I0568399

DISABILITY: AN ANECDOTAL FIELD GUIDE FOR THE REST OF US

A FIELD GUIDE PUBLICATION, VOLUME 1

TRACEE GARNER

GARNER SOLUTIONS, LLC

Acknowledgments

If you don't forsake Lady Wisdom, she will protect you.
Love her, and she will faithfully take care of you.
Gaining sound judgment is key, so first things first: go after Lady Wisdom!
Now, whatever else you do, follow through to understanding.
Cherish her, and she will help you rise above the confusion of life
— your possibilities will open up before you— embrace her, and she will raise you to a place of honor in return.
Proverbs 4:6-8 The Voice

DISABILITY:

AN ANECDOTAL FIELD FOR THE REST OF US, VOLUME 1

Tracee Garner

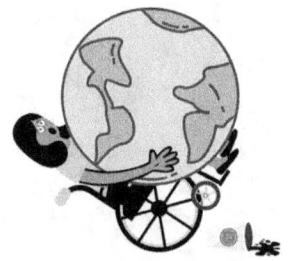

Disability:
An Anecdotal
Field Guide for
the Rest of Us
VOL. I

Disability: An Anecdotal Field Guide for the Rest of Us

© Copyright 2022 by Tracee Garner

www.TraceeGarner.com

Published by Tracee Garner

Ingram Spark Hardcover ISBN: 978-1-957104-20-1

Ingram Spark Ebook ISBN: 978-1-957104-21-8

Formatting by Tracee Lydia Garner

© Editing by Best Words Editing

© Cover Design by Tracee Lydia Garner / Canva

❀ Created with Vellum

INTRODUCTION

Since I was born with Muscular Dystrophy and diagnosed at age two, I've just plain old adapted to this inaccessible life and... well, made it accessible. Well, as much as I can, anyway: you'll have to judge for yourself. But I am a believer that life is what you make it, and I personally feel I've made it very well, thank you.

I have been working on this book for almost 12 years. Now, you may wonder: why on earth did it take so long?

The actual writing took only a few months, but I had to do a couple of things. First, I had to let go of my original vision of the book. You'll learn about what that was in a later chapter – see, if I told you here, you might just skip ahead, you sneaky thing!

Second, I just had to live a lot of stories and take notes to tell you how to be and get along in this life. I know it can be difficult. I know all of the things I'm going to talk about are not easy. I also know you've likely had strife in every sector, but hopefully you learned so much and you are richer for all of those experiences. This may be your first introduction to me and just know this book is a help for the inaccessible ills of life.

The things that make our lives so hard. I'm not here to lament the experience so much, (though I'm sure I will on occasion, it's just human nature) but I am here to help you uncover solutions and keep in your mind ways and means to mitigate all the negative impacts of being a person with a disability. As a long-time advocate for people with disabilities, I get many calls from people seeking help, assistance and guidance. I know just how creative people with disabilities have often had to be, but also how by the time I talk with them they may have exhausted all options.

The very nature of adapting to a relatively inaccessible world means we simply figure everything out for ourselves. With that being said, the truth of this statement is often had by learning from so many others, getting outside ourselves and our world and seeing how others have done it. There is so much to learn from ALL OF US, and in this book, I'm sharing more of the 'what' and 'how' of my own learning in an effort to help you along the journey.

Let's get rolling!

KNOWLEDGE WINS: USING THIS BOOK

I mentioned that it took forever to write this book, right? The thing is, it's been in the works in my head for such a long time, but actually getting around to writing it and narrowing down which topics to tackle in this first offering was another matter. But here we are: in addition to all my other publishing, fiction writing, speaking and teaching projects, as well as working, I finally wrote the thing. I've broken the book down and this is what I have come up with to share with you:

- My own experience in a bite-sized chunk. Yes, the experiences are unique to me, but it's through living it I can tell you what might happen in your life: what I hated about things I faced (which you too may face soon enough); barriers past, present and future; and what you can watch out for as a result, leaning in with the goal in mind so you're ready to meet the issue and hurdle it.
- No two situations are the same, yet people with disabilities throughout my lifetime have generally been treated as the same. Hopefully, with this

resource in hand, you can move through your own
issues on your own path with greater confidence
and maybe get to your level of success just a little
sooner.

- I also talk about what sort of pushback you're likely
to face around the subject, and most importantly,

- I offer a general list of tips and ideas to help you. I'll
always try to provide at least five ideas or tips but in
many sections there are way more than five, in an
effort to help you.

- Finally, you can expect a parting message or
thought with ways you can move forward and
"Take Action."

That's it, really. There is so much more to do after reading
this, but hopefully I will have given you some great ideas to get
you started as well as flagging up some pitfalls to avoid.

A few chapters are longer than others, with more ideas to
take action. Overall, I simply write until it feels like you have
enough information to do something and real make progress. I
don't usually have a set length in mind for my writing, but I also
try not to belabor anything or make it more complex than it has
to be. I want it to be accessible and concise, almost like a reference. I would love it if folks used this as a reference, but it's all
yours: use it however you need and want - and use it, dare I say,
to encourage you and to give you some advance thoughts on
matters you may not yet have considered or needed to tackle.

My final wish is for you to always remember that so much
of this project is about realizing how interconnected and inter-
dependent we all are. One part of disability life is so dependent
on all other parts of disability life. An example of that, for
instance, is the extent to which transportation can get you to

the leisure, recreation and gainful employment that you seek. Where you lack transit and support, your quality of life can be devastatingly affected. Lack of income means you cannot afford transportation, and this affects all other sectors of your life. Case in point.

Finally, thank you so much for purchasing this book. Please write me any time with tips, ideas or just comments. Visit the Garner Solutions, LLC blog for more articles. If you have stories of your own to share, in support of this format of helping others and sharing your own lessons, be sure to read the Your Turn section at the end of the book, and see how you can contribute to Volume Two.

1 / ADVOCACY

KEY TAKEAWAYS

- Look for those who care most for you, your safety and wellbeing. They will teach you your greatest advocacy lessons, and will demonstrate what you need to do as well as how to go about doing it.
- If those that are supposed to care don't rise to the challenge or are not present, trusted surrogates will become vital. People like this do exist: those that stand in but may have no biological relationship to you. Tell them how they can help you and tell them what you want.
- Advocacy is more than just participation in systems that affect your life. It's about the ability to have a personal choice, options and equity.
- Learn components of compelling storytelling, but remember to always tell the truth about how you are treated, how you feel and what you need to be successful. In that truth, powerful people can be compelled and supplied with motivation to take

action on your behalf. If you don't care, why should they?

I credit three resources as the most impactful of all in helping me find my voice. The first two are the state-run programs called Partners In Policymaking (PIP) and the Youth Leadership Forum (YLF-VA). The third, my parents, who were my first demonstration of what advocacy is all about, having to do so at every turn in those early years to ensure I had access to the things I needed.

PIP is a leadership and advocacy training program that teaches individuals with developmental disabilities - and the parents of children with disabilities - to become community leaders and catalysts for systemic change in their local community. While walking this path, participants learn how to obtain the best available services for themselves, their loved ones, and others.

Based on a national model, the overall goal of PIP is to develop productive partnerships between the people who need and use services and those in a position to create policies and laws that affect these services. PIP participants become influencers of change via opportunities to meet and speak with national leaders in the field of developmental disabilities. During class sessions, I would hear presentations about current issues and state-of-the-art practices, as well as policymaking and legislative processes at local, state and national levels.

Both PIP and YLF-VA operate throughout the United States: last I checked, only a few states didn't have the programs available. Their mission was rather simple, and some had anywhere from 5 to 10 important modules that included advocacy, working with your local legislators, and understanding the laws and rights of people with disabilities, as well as an overview of the histories that got us to where we are today. My personal favorite and most impactful component of the programs was understanding how to tell a story.

One of the benefits of the program wasn't just the content but that we - self advocates, which was the category I fit into, about to go into my second year of college at the time - were mixed with parent advocates. I think it was a good idea, all the more so in hindsight, for parents of children with physical and intellectual disabilities to witness the future through me: to see what could be when your parents supported and advocated for you.

My Mom often went with me, but by this time I was up and ready to go to meetings on my own. She had no real interest in the sessions - and, she may argue, I wanted the autonomy of attending events on my own as an independent adult. Trust me, she was plenty happy to stay in the hotel room, order room service, and watch television. It was a win-win. Mom had done this for me most of my later teenage years, but gradually she was realizing that, while I still needed assistance, it was important for me to be able to conduct myself as myself in meetings, with autonomy and independence, and without my mother hanging around all the time. Depending on your age, this transition may be a point of contention. More about that later, but it is important. There are often more parents taking part than self advocates, and it's probably because many self advocates may not have the support to attend.

Finding caregivers to travel for an overnight program is a recurring issue for those of us who require help and support. When I was participating in PIP - and as I know was the case for many similar programs—spending a night or so in a nearby hotel was a requirement. There are all kinds of logistical issues in finding caregivers to travel if you require one. Some state-sponsored programs do assist with some costs, but not all of them and not always.

The second category I've observed is made up of people who simply may not realize how important it is to tell your stories. When you frame your experience in a compelling way, they can help you drive home your points. These stories can be particularly potent when coupled with the benefits of such legislation as the Americans with Disabilities Act (ADA), the Rehabilitation Act, the Olmstead Decision and numerous other civil rights movements. These legal milestones have paved the way for our current level of collective participation in life - this very life you are living! -and continue to permit you access to everything. When you don't know the laws and policies that are specifically designed to help you, you can count on being largely ignored. Those in a position of power will pretend not to know about them unless you speak up.

The only other reason for lack of participation is lack of outreach, as is the case in almost everything for people with disabilities. Outreach to our group has always been an issue of missed opportunities: wasted marketing dollars using the wrong tactics and really failing to understand exactly how people with disabilities access information about community programs and services. In programs like PIP, I was one of so few self-advocates, and until I went through it, I had no idea how important and impactful such a program was going to be. I would argue that at 17 or 18 years of age, you tend to assume those that advocate for you will always be around to do so. We all know that's not the case, but even when we know such things, we still refuse to prepare: parents not only fail to prepare our children for worst-case scenarios, but often actively shield their children from the realities of how hard is to get some of the things they need. The accessible van funds, the extended class time, the reasonable accommodations at school and a plethora of other resources end up being the same types of accommodations needed at work or college - the tutor in college math, for example - and yet these things will need to be had over and over again in different forms, from young adult to older adult settings. Advocacy never ends.

And advocacy is the only thing that changes scenarios.

After participating in nine months of PIP, this advocacy program gave me the tools to speak up and articulate the issues of the day that bothered me. It made me look around and start to see the myriad small infractions happening every day against me, and my friends with disabilities.

I remember such an incident from high school. The Future Business Leaders of America were going on a school trip. A fellow person with a disability was part of the group, but the school did not want to pay for the accessible lift bus to take her. I hated this, but I said nothing. Throughout the years and decades that followed, it has almost felt like karma that transit and lack thereof have seemed like a constant nemesis, out to bother and plague me... until I too advocated for change. The big yellow school bus doesn't work in college, during summer internships and at other milestone moments of adulthood. Had I advocated for my friend back then, would the sheer lack of transportation options and my constant fight for more routes, times and accuracy have remained on my radar for so long? You'll never know for sure, but my point is that the things that constantly reappear in your life somehow tend to be the very issues to which you will find yourself lending your voice: to change systems, ideas, minds, hearts and the humans attached to them.

From the ages of about 18 to 40, I seemed plagued by transit issues. I wouldn't drive until I was in my late twenties because I was denied state financial assistance for my vehicle modifications (extensive hand control system) from someone I now realize was prejudiced against me. He treated the state and federal money as if it were his own personal fund, although it was taxpayer dollars that were there to help me. The bottom line is that the pain points and angst around the issues, as troublesome and depressing as they are, will be the very things that propel you to great action.

It's evident over and over again that whatever issues we initially feel like we can't do anything about or feel voiceless about, we can find our voice as we age or join with others who share similar roadblocks to help amplify all of our voices. The sooner you realize the truth of your parents' limitations and eventual weariness after advocating for you, sometimes for twenty or thirty years of your life and counting, the sooner you understand the critical importance of finding your own voice, learning your needs and uncovering how to be the best advocate you can be for yourself - and for a bunch of others who need you to champion their causes, too.

For as long as I can remember, I have encountered similar issues around not being able to participate: from the church ministry's inaccessible ball game to the ramp at graduation that went up to the stage but not back down on the other side. Yes, the school only wanted to pay for the ramp to go one way. When I got my diploma, it was so awkward and embarrassing to travel back through those waiting in line. You feel dumb: like you're on display as you navigate your way through folks who are focused on listening for their own names. (This particular story made the news, if you can believe that!)

The point is that all these little nicks and cuts and scrapes, seemingly incidental, will become a recurring theme in your life. It's through that constant annoyance and your growing awareness of others' oblivious ignorance that you will find the things you care about.

For some, many of these scenarios will seem so petty, but you might be more likely to relate if you have a high schooler. As insignificant as whatever they want and swear they need is, somehow a parent will find themselves doing all they can to make it happen, because to that teen, it's important, and that also makes it important to you.

Looking back, that two-way ramp wasn't a huge deal, but other things like that - inaccessible events, the loss of social interactions because someone didn't have the forethought to find an accessible venue, poor planning by someone omitting inclusive practices altogether, or the school that says your accessibility needs aren't in the budget - yes, all of that builds up, and when it cuts you one too many times it hurts, plain and simple.

The only way through this is to keep talking, keep advocating, keep pushing back, keep trying, not just in shareable stories like these, but as a recurring theme that will confront you every single day of your life.

As I mentioned, way beyond the state-run programs, the number one best demonstrators of advocacy in motion I've ever encountered would be my Mom and dad. Down at the "school house", as my dad called it, he made sure to make the time to come down and tell all the white ladies gathered around about what I would and would not be doing. When he saw that I wasn't being challenged in my classes, he set about getting me moved out of special education and into general (then called mainstream) education. As I think back now, general education somehow sounded to me like general population: like a prison, where I may have to fend off some real bullies instead of being a top dog in the self-contained special needs class. In case you didn't know, there is a kind of hierarchy among people in the disability community. Sorry to burst your bubble, but it's everywhere. Race, class, gender and ethnic disparities have nothing on the "born with" and "acquired" disability groups. And yes, it's sad. If you haven't yet seen this, you will eventually, and you'll have to chalk it up to being just another crazy thing among human beings.

In essence, this hierarchy says that those who acquire their disability are somehow at odds with those like me who were born with their disability. Or it may be the other way around. It's pure silliness, really, but it does exist. I personally never even recognized it was a thing until I was much older.

As far as my early years, I didn't feel like I wasn't trying. I just never really thought about it, period. It didn't matter enough to me, but looking back, I'm so glad that my parents recognized what was happening and as such took action and got me where I needed to be. This would make all the difference in my future.

I didn't really think of myself as pretending in those special needs classes: only that it didn't seem that hard. Maybe in kindergarten you simply lack ambition: you do color outside the lines, and for most of us, there's not much to strive for when that's acceptable. Yet, I remember being in special education classes, where I stayed until almost the fourth grade.

Being exposed to all these advocacy encounters would ultimately lead me to a point where I would be speaking up for others. Oddly enough, some advocacy was even for caregivers that assisted me. When they found out I wrote books, they would ask me to write things for them: those old government KSAs, letters to their landlord or tenant, or other persuasively worded letters for the purpose of getting something, getting out of something or getting something resolved. This opened my eyes to the fact that advocacy can be not only the spoken word, but the written word as well.

I was just wordy, verbose and direct in written form. Sometimes that also got me in trouble. Later, at about sixteen years of age, I can remember starting to write my own letters for everything. Applying for the DMV placard (which I don't think you have to do anymore) to show proof of disability, recommendation letters, accommodation letters, requests, policy drafts... In every sector where I needed permission or support for a program or recommendation, I was the one who wrote the letter. For medical issues, I would often write the letter then ask my doctor to sign it, and the deed was done. I was pretty excited to start driving, but because I had to have extensive hand controls, I was required to do a six-page medical report every two or three years! I never want to lose my driving privileges, I thought, but what if at some point I missed this two-year re-up? After considering this, I wrote a letter explaining that I know when I'm sick and that I would never put others in danger, so could I please be excused from periodically proving my ability?

All of this taught me that you simply never know unless you try. I didn't run it by anyone. I didn't ask whether it was a good idea. I've always said, "let me try". What if my dad hadn't determined that I would do better in 'general population' school? I can never remember hearing my parents discuss any pushback or even an outright no, denying my access. Back then, he likely heard: "What does he know? He's not a teacher." But my dad knew me, he knew what I was capable of, and he also knew that without some pushing, I probably wouldn't rise to the occasion. All of this may have been so, but he didn't back down. We all should be confident enough to do the same.

Writing and speaking weren't overly important to me per se, but it was the only way I believed things were going to get done in a timely fashion, maybe even change. I also found them to be the best ways of honestly saying the things I wanted to say and framing my own story. Most of the time, I was only asking others to endorse it. I learned that when I presented information and arguments to them in a compelling way, they did exactly that, and continued to do so to this day.

At some point, you'll have to take a stance and let others know what's right for you. It's about control - about having a say in what happens - but equally it's about dignity and respect. At all times, you should have a clear idea of what exactly it is you want and need to live your life. No one should you deter you from making that happen; and only you will know what needs to be said in your specific situation. Look it up and see what has already been said throughout history, then build on that with the aim of getting further than those before you. State your case, then never accept "no" as a final answer. Keep trying, get their endorsement and bring others along with you.

Currently, 35 states have Partners In Policymaking programs. The core values largely state similar objectives across all programs, in that:

- People with disabilities are people, first. We are not "the handicapped" or "the disabled." Using People-First Language is a must.
- People with disabilities need real friendships, not just relationships with paid staff.
- People with disabilities are entitled to the full meaning of The First Amendment right to free speech. The ability to communicate, in whatever

form, must be available to every person with a disability.

- People with disabilities must be able to enjoy full mobility and accessibility that allows active participation in community life.
- People with disabilities must be assured continuity in their lives through families and neighborhood connections.
- People with disabilities must be treated with respect and dignity.
- People with disabilities need to be in positions to negotiate to have their wants and needs met.
- People with disabilities must be able to exercise choice in all areas of their lives.
- People with disabilities must be able to live in the homes of their choices with the supports they need; and
- People with disabilities must be able to enjoy the benefits of true productivity through employment and/or contributions as members of their communities, and
- People with disabilities must be able to enjoy the benefits of true productivity through employment, volunteerism, and/or other ways to offer our contributions as full members of their communities.

- A child's primary caregiver and those he/she spends the most time with will be the largest influence on them, and that means you have power for how they will relate (or not) to everything.
- I would argue that teaching advocacy can be had at just the months old mark for any child, with teaching kids to ask outright (or using some form of language to inform their parents, or others, of their needs, even non-verbal). It does not matter the method; it matters that someone can learn to understand and the child can learn to not only be heard but understand they must do a single act to propel others to action, even if that simple action is needing water or other sustenance.
- Never be afraid to offer correction. Not everything your child will do is appropriate and will result in positive reinforcement or reward. It can't be solely a reward system. This is not the real world. See what they want before offering everything through conversation and negotiation with time. This will

help with getting them to the things they need through push and pull mechanics of diplomacy and compromise.

- Always be questioning. The best way to gauge where your child/youth/young adult is at one subject is to just ask. These may be issues they've seen in the course of a day, the day's headlines, news and find the time to look up pending legislation and policy, particularly ones that pertain to disability, civil, race, reproductive, gender and human rights. Talk about current rules and regulations and how it may or may not affect them and others like them.

- Don't deny your children the opportunity to participate in things away from you/away from home. These experiences build confidence. One example is that there is a certain vocational rehabilitation venue that contains both young adults with behavioral issues related to their disabilities and those with disabilities brought on by substance abuse issues. There is no judgment in either the why or how these groups came to be. My point is that in helping make parents a determination in whether or not to send their child to this facility, it is important for them to consider NOT the facility and it's issues but the child and what is their level of self-autonomy. While this might seem horrifying to consider, kids are around all types of people on a daily basis in the community; in a closed, contained venue, some kids can attend the week, or month long cohort, returning to home life fine, while others are not ready to be in this environment, easily duped, manipulated, coerced and sometimes irrevocably pressured into bad behavior. As scary as this might sound, there are things you can do to ensure you know whether or not this can be option for your child prior to signing off on their participation. One way is to often, offer your children different scenarios to gauge their response to matters as well as their resourcefulness. If you need to set up scenarios in a controlled environment, do that. You will know exactly what your child is capable of and identify weak spots for bad behavior and worst-case situations before they can occur. No test is perfect. That is absolutely true, but having some sense of where your child is at mentally and emotionally can help you know what programs they should and should not participate in. A week long camp, a day-support program, or a day camp are all good short-term programs that can strengthen your child's ability, and so many parents in an effort to protect their child may find themselves denying opportunities to participate, which is not at all helpful either. You want your child, eventually, to be able to get along without you and expose them to different people and scenarios without you there to rescue them.

- Do not attend meetings without your child present unless absolutely necessary. Children, even if coloring, or you've given them something to occupy them and keep them quiet, can still be in the room because they ARE STILL LISTENING and WATCHING THE BODY LANGUAGE OF

YOU and OTHERS IN THE ROOM. Both your body language and how you handle things and that of others in a position of authority, e.g., their teachers, therapist, counselor and others. I would suggest that having your child present could have a positive effect in that you might be willing to fight a little harder and, in the cases of some IEP meetings, you may work even that much more not to succumb to your emotions such as crying or yelling simply because you don't want to exhibit that kind of behavior for your child to witness. While these meetings are extremely volatile and schools often come across as bullies, seemingly pitting parents simply trying to advocate for their child's needs against decision makers who come off as doing whatever they can to withhold everything from you and your child. It should not be such a marred and emotionally charged space but unfortunately though all parties have what's best for the child, it comes down to what they are and are not willing to pay for to make that happen, (and yes, who has more resources and lawyers to ultimately win). That's unfortunate. Arm yourself with knowledge. There are classes you can take. Use what you've learned from your day job and the business world about negotiation tactics and influencing others. Where funding is an issue, find your own funding sources in the form of grants and scholarships for therapies and treatment programs. Apply, apply, apply. There are a number of programs that are available until your child is eighteen. Those programs often dry up as your child ages, making them no longer eligible regardless of financial need. Lastly, fundraise. Many campaigns through popular crowd funding platforms can work for you and other families for a good cause. Should you have to do this, no, but to get your child the things he/she needs, you may have to and it can mean everything between success, access and inclusion or failure.

- Practice making statements of need and help your child to craft these statements, periodically practicing so they are ready to go at any opportunity they are asked to speak up.

2 / EMPLOYMENT

Key Takeaways

- You will have to push back against naysayers every single day and at every stage of life. "They say" will never stop.
- Regarding the temptation to blame others for your employment results: As well as frequently defending your own knowledge, skills and abilities, you'll have to challenge your own negative, self-effacing beliefs that can be the real robbers of success. You'll also need to come to terms with the fact that many people in hiring positions maintain unfortunate and wrong ideas about the training, hiring and retention of people with disabilities. Getting past some of these may require professional assistance - hiring a coach, for example - as well as thinking outside the traditional employment box.
- While there are federally funded vocational

rehabilitation centers in almost every state to assist you with your employment goals, such resources can only be as good as your own advocacy efforts and your own willingness to be proactive in your quest for gainful employment.

- Dabble in EVERYTHING. There is no greater way to find what you enjoy than sampling something on the ENTIRE buffet.

The one thing I strongly dislike (read: hate) about disability's impact on my professional life is that society tends to stick people with disabilities in boxes according to a case manager's perception, historical data or societal norms dictating what we can do, rather than listening to our own desires and goals. Rare is the conversation that is centered on what we want to do, not just what we are qualified for – usually only physically, at that.

You might be surprised to know that I feel I got this question wrong when I interviewed for a job with a Center for Independent Living. I didn't realize it at the time. There was a question about what I would do in a situation where someone wanted to work at ABC company and they had a certain disability, asking how I would work with them or the course of action I would recommend. (In my defense, and for those of us who still hold limiting beliefs, it was something like a dancer for a person with Down Syndrome.)

I bombed it.

I had no idea about disability from a case management and independent-living-philosophy mindset at that time, and there really wasn't much training available about it. Of course I know it now. My response was something akin to getting the person with a disability as close as possible to their desired job: in the same building, perhaps, or in an administrative role, with the hope that they could move forward at some point in the future. To be frank, I thought it seemed like a ridiculous case scenario. The bottom line, and what the hiring officials were after, was that at the end of the day, the purpose of the role for which I was interviewing was to facilitate the person getting the job they wanted, come what may. If it didn't happen, okay - but I was to do whatever was in my power to help them reach their own goal.

I actually wasn't hired at my first attempt. A few years later I applied again, equipped by that time with the knowledge that just because you don't know every historical detail about disability and the movement doesn't mean you can't be a relevant, productive and staunch advocate for others.

For me, what it took to truly understand this was simply to have a few more limitations put on my own goals. Being told what I should do, rather than having what I wanted to do acknowledged, definitely helped me to understand how much getting in line with folks' desires is the best course of action. Perhaps there was also some level of fear around my abilities to help, coupled with some existing real-world knowledge that it often isn't the applicant's lack of determination and willingness that stops them, but rather outright refusals from those in positions of power. Taken together, this would suggest that it's also productive to help others manage their expectations. Ultimately, it's about accepting a hard dose of what society unfortunately still gets wrong about capability and human potential.

After the fact, of course, it seemed such a no-brainer. Realizing my error yet trying to show compassion to myself, I had to remind myself that in answering that question the way I did, I was simply referring back to my own experience. As had been done to me, my first instinct was to place limitations on another based on my own preconceptions about ideal work and placement for them. That being said, how can anyone help someone else to do something that they themself haven't seen in practice? This is why so many people with disabilities lament the lack of images of themselves on television. There may certainly be someone out there with a disability that has attained the level of success and satisfaction that you crave and hope to obtain at some point, but how do you stay motivated if you don't ever see images of these success stories publicized and celebrated?

In the same way, I became aware that I never see images of African-American folks with disabilities in loving, long term relationships. The African-Americans I saw were invariably folks who were originally nondisabled when they married, then had been confronted by accident or injury only later and further along the path of their relationship. Do you see the issue with this? I realize it can difficult to stay in relationships when a partner has been injured, but folks often do *because the love has already been established.* You're already invested in that person, so you're not building a relationship with a disabled person from scratch.

Back to that essay I was asked to write for that job application. Knowing nothing about the independent living movement and having few to no models of what I should do, I had to begin the process of wrapping my head around the concept of people with various kinds of disabilities in other kinds of roles.

As a woman in my forties, I personally feel that I'm pretty self-aware. I'm in touch with the issues and the figurative baggage around disability that we often pick up and carry. I did not want another person with a disability to run into the devastating feelings that can come with outright rejection. At some point, though, you will inevitably start to weigh some of your experiences and your willingness to try through the lens of rejection. The same is true in relationships, as well as in making the decision to work. Some people with disabilities believe the stressors and the judgment are simply too great to risk venturing into an employment setting. You may think this is not true: that anyone who wants to work can do so, and that anyone who doesn't work simply doesn't want to. I'm here to tell you that's not true. Some can and some physically cannot, but any and all of the following could be at play:

- **Judgment**. Consider a person who has put in twenty-five years at a company, then has a stroke or a medical setback. Rather than letting them return to work after rehabilitation, coworkers may start a mill of exaggerations, untruths and whispers about his or her abilities, implying that the job can no longer be performed by said person. Such whispers are often not true. There may be ways to modify schedules, there may be supports or modifications to the workspace that could be made. In fact, in an application for social security, it's one of the questions they ask you: Have you made efforts to modify the job? Such efforts aren't for the employee to make alone, however, but for the employee and the employer to come up with possible solutions together. Yes, as an employee you should explore all available resources and think about ways to approach the problem, but an employer should likewise be willing and ready to entertain possible methods to resolve issues. Instead, he or she has often moved onto the next person, all too ready to let that first person go.

- Lack of accommodation and support to provide reasonable accommodation to people with disabilities in the workplace - even when it is the law. When you're made to feel 'less than', who would then have the emotional and mental wherewithal to submit the paperwork for the things they need? Especially knowing that upon submission, you'll face scrutiny when other colleagues find out about your requests (because nothing is truly confidential). Don't dismiss your own suffering in that kind of scenario. Remaining at home and collecting a check is a fine, honest and legal option, although sadly, it's what society expects - regardless of the fact that the check in question is sadly not enough for most people to live on.

- **Perception of others**. These 'others' may be of the opinion that you're not disabled at all, or perhaps that your required supports costs them money personally. Such people may misguidedly think that giving to you what you ask for poses a threat to their bottom line, or their salary, or their overtime. Many a manager has acted like the accommodation budget is their own discretionary fund and, as the gatekeeper of such a resource, they can't possibly spare the dollars for, say, elevated foot plates for the little person; an electric desk that raises and lowers for the person who uses a wheelchair; the ergonomic chair with lumbar support; automatic doors, or a ramp... and on and on and on. This attitude persists despite the myriad federal dollars, grants, programs and even tax incentives in place to incentivize an employer to follow to the law and provide these necessary remedies.

The scenarios I've outlined may sound extreme, but they are all taken from life: real instances I've either heard about or personally witnessed.

When I think about self-awareness, it's about waking up to the existence of a continued stigma against people with disabilities being a presence in the workplace.

Whenever I work on Social Security applications, which is often, it's never that that person cannot work, it's that those in positions of power refuse to hire. That is both the tragedy and the battle.

When I think about what I wrote in that application essay, I always think: 'Hey, at least I wrote about *trying*.' At least I envisioned a strategy to get them even a little closer to their desired profession, just hoping for a little right-time-right-place luck to do the rest. Hoping, as ever, that someone would see the determination - that there'd be even one open-minded person who'd see what people with disabilities could do, rather than their frequent focus on all that we can't...

We have to daily confront our own belief in our abilities. We'll often have to prove what we're capable of. And yes, we'll have to brace ourselves for perpetual rejection without so much as an opportunity to demonstrate our capabilities, and this will be a deterrent for many. It is hard to set up meeting after meeting with those who offer token interviews, knowing all the while that your resume is headed for the circular file as soon as you leave their office. But, regardless, you have to. You have things to contribute. You are knowledgeable, and you can share your talents with others. While the allure of even a few dollars coming automatically from the government can be tempting, it won't ever truly get you the things you need in life, in any sense. Trust me.

In all the Myers Briggs type indicator tests, as well as just about every other personality test or quiz there was, writing didn't come up for me. My first job at sixteen was through the placement of a work program, and later the Workforce Development Program. These hands-on experiences were key. Another thing that disability can limit is all those sports opportunities. No basketball, soccer or other contact sport where children really develop some of their likes and dislikes. Still, try to get into as many different kinds of opportunities for work and other interaction that you and your parents can find. More than any aptitude test, this is the real way to zero in on what you do and don't like: to truly identify your passions.

While I was never necessarily qualified to be a writer, it was something that I worked at and that I liked. What do we say to English and Art Majors? It doesn't pay; the only jobs are teaching position which – you guessed it - doesn't pay. What I've learned that it may be true, depending on what you end up doing, that it doesn't pay a lot - but *it does pay* and it is a way to make a living. Not to mention the immeasurable extra benefits to be had if you like what you're doing, let alone if there is a vestige of sanity to be had at the end of the day. Isn't that in itself a significant part of the pay packet? It pays: not always in dollars, but it does make sense.

As you make your way to your chosen employment vocation, you'll want to be sure you've tried every possible thing that you could. In that trying and testing and testing and trying, you'll find what resonates with you and what you love most.

Don't be afraid to build a career around the discoveries you make. Even if there is just one related profession, you at least know there is one; if there are many, as I've found to be the case with writing, there are many. From my own work and my own canvassing have come a number of options that, when pieced together, make up a career and a life. And no-one has the right to say what that should or should not be.

My Mom brings up a particular little article that I wrote in elementary school that should have been a sign of my future as a writer. I do also remember a short story or two, but to be honest it wasn't on my radar, period. What I did notice was that speaking up for myself and articulating my thoughts really made me feel powerful, so I did run with it. In life, you often become a storyteller out of necessity, in order to get the things you need and the access you're frequently denied - in order to bring people around to your way of thinking.

I'm excited and hopeful for today's inclusive practices, represented by the fact that the majority of children are no longer bussed, as I was. I remain optimistic that perhaps full integration can began to set in and take hold. Your non-disabled child may be fully integrated with a child or two that are on the spectrum, and depending on your response, the possibility of full integration is there. We can begin to see and grow with folks who don't always look or learn like us. As this attitude becomes a more expected part of life, perhaps the next generations will develop the ability to remove more of the old stigmas and blinders. Maybe one day, when today's and tomorrow's children are in a position to hire, it won't be a big deal at all. They will relate to and see the people that they grew up with and went to school with, and will thus be more likely to find ways to make it all work - instead of producing the usual pathetic variety of excuses, as referenced above, for why it won't.

Already, our next generations of people with disabilities have conquered almost every employment sector, from dancing, broadcasting and acting to modeling for major fashion brands such as Target. Mattel has a number of Barbie Fashionista dolls representing people with prosthetic limbs, as well as people with viligo, alopecia and/or cancer represented by a Barbie that's bald, plus a number of other disabilities. Such dolls could really help children who aren't accustomed to seeing such images reflecting themselves; or help non-disabled children encounter such differences more naturally, as nothing to be afraid of.

Still, it's clear that even toys have accessibility battles to face. Share a Smile Becky, the wheelchair-using Barbie, doesn't fit into the Dream House, and there is not a single elevator. Hopefully all this will soon be remedied, though. I have a feeling that Becky and her new friends are great advocates.

A Word on Creative Endeavor As Gainful Employment Opportunity

We're so fortunate that within the last fifteen years, creative entrepreneurial ventures have really been able to take off online. Most notably, since the dawn of Etsy and eBay in 2005, creatives of all stripes can now work with a "storefront" shop online featuring brilliant photos and descriptions, all while remaining relatively unseen themselves.

Now, before anyone takes issue with that, let me be clear: I'm not saying we should ever hide. I'm simply saying that in a world that is not always accepting, some desire this anonymity to avoid potentially painful judgment and shunning attitudes: the very factors that may have held them back from working in traditional roles in the first place. Of course, yes, it's incumbent upon every individual to see themselves in a way that's positive and to constantly demonstrate that you can contribute to society no matter your predisposition, but that doesn't mean the negativity does not hurt. It's exhausting. Too much of it slowly and painfully pushes some folks into their homes: the only place they feel safe from judging eyes.

Ceaseless commentary, said in person or online; shaming memes with unflattering photos put up for more views, using still more deeply hurtful language. I talked about that in this chapter. Even as someone who fits the definition of what society deems "normal looking" (minus the wheelchair), I've still felt the brunt of silent stares when the ramp on my accessible vehicle deploys, quickly making my independence feel about as normal and natural as a second head. I've encountered the folks who won't assist me at the grocery store because they feel I should have thought to bring my own assistance - a caregiver or parent, perhaps (never a spouse, mind you: that would just be crazy), or that maybe I should have just stayed home altogether. Don't get it twisted: the majority of folks are willing, but you might be familiar with that look on a cashier's face that says "I'm tired and I don't bag anymore" – the person who'll call the lowest person on the totem pole to help. This is still out there and it occurs more often than I care to admit. This may sound awfully extreme. I wish it weren't. It is changing, for sure. Everything is *changing all the time, for both the better and the worse; but for some, the damage has already been done.*

So, yes, in a world of ever-increasing online consumption with owners/creators increasingly unseen, it can be a huge boon that your product can now go before you. With an attractive and well-maintained website, a person with a disability can earn an income. This has become the way for many entrepreneurial minds to earn a solid, honest and purposeful living. Side hustles and creative endeavors are great ways to do something you love, yet these creative outlets could be so much more than side hustles. People with disabilities could benefit most from it, owing to the simple fact that the hiring managers can't seem to be persuaded to hire more of us. We need to spread the word and teach those that could most use this alternative, nontraditional way to attain income online. This option could be an accessible and lucrative way to pursue the things and projects that you like to do in the comfort and privacy of your home, and there is nothing at all wrong with that.

TAKE ACTION ON EMPLOYMENT

- Do you know your rights when it comes to disability disclosure in an employment setting, or during the interview process?
- When an employer asks about the nature of your disability, what will you say? Never mind the fact that they are not supposed to ask you under the disclosure policy. They may or may not know this. Regardless, HOW you handle it can make or break your entire interview, even if they are in fact in the wrong.
- How will you address questions about your work and gaps in work history (which may or may not be due to disability)?
- Find ten of the hardest questions and prepare/practice your response to them. Practice in the mirror. Are you angry? Do you appear confident in your response? Are there nervous tics that give away how you are really feeling?
- Realize that your morale around employment is something that you need to deal with. This has

nothing to do with your ability but with the fact that societal barriers remain. However, it affects you tremendously and will have a significant bearing on your ability to feel good, day in and day out, in your quest for gainful employment opportunities. You may need to stop looking or to take a day off. You may need to chat with others, not just other job seekers in general but specifically to other job seekers with disabilities, as we are the ones who can truly understand the unique barriers that we face.

- Take a break.
- Consider consulting an employment coach or a nonprofit that assists people with finding a job. Nonprofits in your area will have connections. Completing their intake process, or going through an orientation if applicable, can help you identify problem areas where you may even be shooting yourself in the foot.
- Have your resume overhauled professionally to ensure you are making the most of that piece of paper.
- Talk to an image consultant. Yes, as a person with a disability, there may be things that no amount of clothing, makeup or Spanx can hide, but there may be some aspects of your personal presentation, such as dirty glasses or even word choice, that speak volumes and that you can do something about if you're just made aware of them.
- Nonprofits can also conduct mock interviews (you can also try this with a trusted friend.) This exercise can offer vital feedback to help you make

improvements. Recording such sessions is also a good idea, to help you catch points of hesitation and other things you cannot identify or address in real time during the mock session. If working with a friend, ask them for their honest critiques, too.

- How will you respond to the tough questions? Write them down and practice your answers.
- Ensure federally funded employment / ticket to work and incentive programs are making progress and giving you viable offers. If they seem insistent on only offering you retail, data entry or low-level customer service employment opportunities, consider the reasons. Is this really a result of your knowledge and skill inventory, or might some old thinking held by the case manager be the real culprit in the types of positions they return for you?
- While placement will be more difficult for some types of disabilities over others, you nonetheless have to be a stellar candidate and exhaust ALL resources.
- Can you get a certificate in a special skill/competency, perhaps at a trade school or through an apprenticeship or volunteer opportunity? These can be promising options if time, money and/or learning capabilities do not allow entry to extended education degree programs.
- Until you are sure about what you want, TRY EVERYTHING! Take the personality tests, but be careful not to let them put you in a box of limited options for possible professions.
- Look to other supports beyond your local

organizations and nonprofits. Resource centers are statewide, regionally funded services, and online programs are also cropping up. I personally like Mercedes Swan, specializing in millennial job assistance; there are resources there and at Flex Jobs, specifically geared toward remote work opportunities. I repeat: TRY EVERYTHING.

- LOOK FOR OPPORTUNITIES: don't just let them come to you.

- Take the personality type quizzes. There's a wide range of options out there: the old standard Myers-Briggs Type Indicator (MBTI); the Dominance, Influence, Steadiness, and Compliance (DISC) Assessment; Interpersonal Skills assessment; Sokanu career assessment tool. There's also the more in-depth Enneagram, focusing more on your personality as a whole and how it affects your handling of various issues. These tools are not the be all and end all, but they can be helpful in assisting you with exploring which things you like most. Granted, I may just enjoy taking quizzes of self-discovery, but I urge you to realize how much insight they offer. And you don't have to be religious to take the Spiritual Gifts class that I enjoyed at my local church, having not even known that they offered such a thing. Remember, however, that while these are helpful tools, you shouldn't let them pigeon hole you into limited options. They should be coupled with other tools and outlets for self-awareness and discovery. None of these tools are the last word about who you are, nor are they necessarily any indication of what you'll excel or fail at, nor thus the best fitting job opportunities. Although they make an attempt to tackle the endless subtleties of personality, these tests still fall far short of the real deal: you!

- When results from the aforementioned type indicator are returned, look through ALL of them, NOT just the ones that are "physically doable" for your physical capabilities.
- Write down what you want, including a mix of different aspects of what you would like to do: what kind of employer you want, what kind of environmental setting would be ideal, even management styles.
- Realize you cannot get all of those things, but highlight or star the non-negotiable.
- If you're going to work with an organization that is supposed to assist people with disabilities in their quest for employment, be hands-on and proactive. Don't simply expect them to return a list of possible jobs back to you each week.
- Stay on top of the organization, advocate for yourself, but realize the role you yourself play in your success.
- Ensure service providers have built relationships with employers (as is their job.)
- See what other clients have to say. Don't let the fact that they receive government funding deter you from exploring their track record. In fact, hold them accountable when you don't get the results you feel you are entitled to. At the same time, don't forget to manage your own expectations, too.

- Work with as many service providers as possible, not just a single agency.
- If you feel the jobs they return are not in line with what you want, at least be willing to try it, before concluding that it's somehow "beneath" you - or whatever ill feelings you have about the proposed positions.
- Do not let the fact that you may not be applying for a federal job deter you from seeking resume review and enhancement help.

3 / MENTAL HEALTH

KEY TAKEAWAYS

- Disability can complicate matters around mental health, but there is help available that can speak to the challenges you have despite the added layers of complexity.
- Stigma around mental health support should never deter you from seeking professional help.
- Look beyond the mental health practitioners to peers and older adult figures with similar disabilities, same gender identification and other personal attributes to further support you in understanding and dealing with your issues, as they too have had to face what you are dealing with. While folks in similar situations can be a resource, also be aware that having a shared disability experience shouldn't be the only consideration. Remain conscious that this doesn't automatically create a shared way of thinking about issues and topics.

- The most important qualities are sound advice, reliability, and empathy for your experience, regardless of whether or not you share similar challenges or situations.

While we all process things differently, we can likely agree that if you've ever had an opportunity to meet and talk with a licensed professional counselor of some sort, for any issue, it has been beneficial to you at that particular stage in life.

Around my late twenties, early thirties, I found myself needing to speak with a counselor. Searching for a sense of place, employment, relationship: these things felt extra weighty and extra burdensome with a disability.

At the time, I was getting older. My chronic condition meant that I was experiencing weakened muscles and some increased physical limitations that to me were extremely depressing. While my mind was sharp and fast, my body - limbs, stamina and strength - just would not cooperate with my mental ability. These issues are difficult when you do not have a disability, so having one as well can complicate the layers of processing.

I will say briefly that in every area of life I've lived so far, issues tend to crop up around disability in five particular areas. This does not apply to everyone, but when I feel a sense of needing to run - or roll! - away from the issues, these usually stem from disability in the following areas:

A FAILED RELATIONSHIP

A BROKEN DREAM or MISSED (supposedly "GOLD-EN") OPPORTUNITY

FEELING CHAINED, BOXED IN or LIMITED BY PHYSICAL CHAINS (i.e. a lack of strength, inaccessibility to participate, feeling 'less than' or lacking independence)

DISAPPOINTMENT BY PEOPLE, ESPECIALLY THOSE THAT CLAIM TO CARE THE MOST FOR YOU

The reason I mention these things is that if you feel a sense of any of the above, it's important for you get to the root cause – sometimes referred to as 'triggering' - that creates a downward spiral, potentially leading to depression.

As an older, mature woman, I can now recognize that resistance or even failings in these areas cause great and unnecessary adversity. I recognize them now, but also realize that I can make a choice to do the work to overcome those things.

One example of this from my own experience took place over what I've come to call The Covid Summer. It was that notorious summer of 2020 when a caregiver of mine left abruptly without notice. I was so angry: down in the dumps, depressed and relating everything back to disability. You know the drill:

Why me?

Why do I always need help?

Why do I have to be disabled?

Why can't I have a little added strength to at least _____ (insert whatever you can't do but would like to be able to do, e.g. transfer, stand, bear weight) myself?

Why did this happen?

Why does my body betray me?

The actions of others have absolutely nothing to do with me. People will move on and this will often be hard to accept, but it happens in all sorts of relationships. You are free to mourn your relationship that has been lost, but you cannot give up on yourself.

Each and every time I hire and train a new aide, the chore is the training. As with any new employee, it can be a challenge getting them acclimated to assisting me and knowing my personal needs, but eventually they learn, they are there for you and you are able to move on from the one that didn't work out before.

Having someone in your corner, several folks in fact, is key in coping when these pitying questions crop up. Back then, I had my bestie, also a person with a disability, who understood what it was like to experience the constant turnover of caregiver support. Our shared understanding made it easier to get through and to talk with her about.

Having a counselor who helped me realize that it's not a personal thing when folks move on was also helpful. Just being able to freely vent was important, too. My bestie was also the first person I know who used Craigslist to find her potential applicants. I had personally been afraid of this platform: probably a result of having watched the *Craigslist Killer* movie on Lifetime several years ago. An important caveat: when I finally started tentatively using Craigslist myself, it was only with lots of precautions. There are many actions you can take to protect yourself and your identity, so please be cautious. Before using any social platform, you must learn the necessary steps you should take to protect yourself. Please see a special course I offer on hiring caregivers prior to doing anything like this.

After all my caution prior to my first posting, I was pleasantly surprised by the number and caliber of folks who inquired about the position.

As far as my own experience goes, however, disability always felt like such a hindrance. Yet, I'm well aware that to folks outside your inner circle, you look and appear completely independent. If you're anything like me, your disposition is rather calm - happy-go-lucky, even - and you exhibit a great deal of optimism in spite of your condition. This is what folks have always told me about how I live my life with a disability.

All of that may be true, but there can be times where you're confronted by your limitations. When most able-bodied people's car breaks down, it's straightforward to call someone to get a ride and off you go: Uber or Lyft or a cab. Those things are just not always accessible to folks who cannot walk or stand. Not all wheelchairs fold into separate lightweight, manageable pieces that fit into a compact car's trunk. These are just some of the things that you have to find ways around. Getting stuck waiting for transportation - much like experiencing illness, obtaining employment, having an intimate relationship – is rendered much more complex by the nature of your disability. It increases your medical bills, requires specialized transportation, triggers added wait times, stigma, stares by others; and that's not to mention the costly equipment needed simply to live your life and get around. All of that can weigh on you and make you feel exasperated by the level of coordination and logistical planning required just to get up and get where you are going. Anyone who tells you it's not taxing is, quite frankly, just too happy.

I'm expressing all of this to say that if you need it, or you feel overwhelmed by all that is involved with disability life, there is help available, and there is absolutely nothing wrong with seeking support. I'm here to tell you that such support makes all the difference, coming alongside you not just to listen but also to provide ideas, new thinking and new ways of handling situations. I also count it as a wonderful privilege to have had the healthcare coverage to allow me to find and pay someone to render such aid.

Psychologists can't diagnose, but they offer so much more. I was fully aware that the professionals I saw could not prescribe medication, and that was how I wanted it. For many folks, it won't be about medications: it will be about talking out the things that bother you, then talking more, and doing a bit of listening as well, all to work though the situation.

Finally, sometimes there is no solution, or the solution isn't what you want to hear.

I remember telling a family member how I wished I didn't need help. I was annoyed with their response: a sad, pitying face that essentially said, "Yeah, okay, but you do." My response might have been: "Thank you, Captain Obvious." I was annoyed with the face that reminded me once again of something of which I'm already painfully aware. That is precisely what people with disabilities don't need. When you ask for reasonable accommodation, you don't need to be told that it costs extra, that plans might need to be altered, that this and that need to be moved to accommodate your disability. *Over and over again.* These are not helpful, empathetic responses. Some responses essentially tell you to suck it up: that ultimately, this isn't something you should be upset over at all.

Bear in mind that others don't get to decide what is and is not worth feeling for you. You are the only one that can decide a course of action and how to deal with something. You have to assess what you need. It could be as simple as talking to someone, or multiple people, such as a support group - another great resource for group strategy, with more ideas being added to the common pot of solutions by so many folks sharing their similar experience; or one person to talk to, or medication, or therapies, or treatment. *You* decide, then you set about doing and getting what you need. There is no right or wrong; there is no single answer.

Counseling offers an opportunity to be heard, to share whatever you want, and to receive or be offered ideas about what to do to cope and create change. You may see someone for a prolonged period of time, you may see someone for just a few months, maybe a year. For me, it was a chance to release the problems as I saw them. While everything obviously could not be solved, having someone repeat your own ideas back to you, hear you and help you work through your problems can be the best kind of help. When we are stuck in our own minds about things, this is to our detriment. The mind often offers only solutions that are readily available and obviously doable. Solutions gained through meeting and talking with others may stretch your definition of "doable" and challenge you to grow and try new things.

I don't currently see anyone but, having had such a great experience the first time, I'm open to it and ready if ever I feel the need arise. Moreover, when my best friend - whom I would talk to often and who had a similar disability to mine - passed away in 2019, it definitely left a void. That being said, her passing also made me realize that a) I would have to venture out to find and connect with new friends who had similar disabilities; and b) that would take time, commitment and work.

I mentioned another resource where I have found good information but wasn't quite for me: local support groups. People experiencing what you are experiencing are some of the best people to help you. They can understand how you feel and that makes a difference. People with similar disabilities to your own often won't trivialize or discount worries you express. They will have tried similar remedies, thus living by example to know what to tell you to do. It's really an almost instant referral network for doctors, lawyers, therapists, dentist, other medical practitioners, drugs (consult your doctor first of course), even supplements and holistic remedies. What I loved was being able to ask where the heck to get durable medical equipment repaired, along with numerous other topics that would crop up.

If a counselor is not for you, then the support of others with similar conditions could be what you need and truly beneficial in the long run.

Other areas that people might have issues around are trauma, situations they can't escape from, financial, emotional and more. Obviously, if you have dealt with trauma, an experienced professional is vital and you should seek whatever you need to deal with that.

When I mention the categories where mental health support is needed on the previous pages, I do so because I have personally seen a large number of breakdowns and mental upset around loss: the loss of someone; the loss of a relationship; moving or relocation; the loss of the things that are dignifying, such as employment; tragic and sudden death; setbacks in physical and mental health; and family or caregiver-related stress. In the last few years, this has been underpinned by the widespread images of injustice, violence and brutality against marginalized persons. I'm not saying there aren't significantly more things than this, just that these are the top recurring events that create upset within the mind and infiltrate our thought processes, causing a downward spiral if we do not seek attention about it.

I haven't had to see anyone since that time, but I am now always evaluating whether or not I should and won't hesitate to do so if the time comes.

Regarding my counselor, I know that one important thing for me was to find someone outside my personal and local circles. I realize that gossip and whisperings about people and their "issues" are one of the unfortunate reasons folks do not seek the help they need, and that is tragic. What I did to mitigate this occurrence was simply to go to a larger organization than what was in my backyard or where I was already attending for my worship services. This cut down the possibility that I'd run into someone I knew coming out of the same office and thus gave me more anonymity – although that can still happen, of course. I offer this as an example and another option, thanks to the availability of telehealth appointments prevalent in the pandemic. Research places such as Talk or Better Help, along with other popular platforms, where you can find support without leaving the comfort of your own home.

Despite wanting your dealings to remain private from others and your professional and personal social networks, we can't let the possibility of seeing someone you know in your circles, deter you from seeking help for yourself. I encourage you that your own demonstration of honesty, your bravery even, could help push someone else to get help for themselves and continue breaking the stigma and the cycle of shame associated with mental health counseling.

TAKE ACTION ON MENTAL HEALTH

- While this chapter has been largely about counseling, support groups and peers with disabilities, first take a look at your situation. WHO is your trusted tribe? Do you have one? Do you need to first identify a small group of positive supporters? A network?
- When you think about seeking counseling, what has prevented you from moving forward with it?
- What research do you need to do?
- What topics would you talk about if you had a meeting right now?
- What kinds of comments, either in passing or when conversing directly, has your family expressed about counseling?
- Where might you look to find someone?
- Would a support group be something to try first? (Many support groups are free through mental health organizations, hospitals, faith-based groups, addiction and recovery programs, but contain folks who have similar issues, however are also largely

unsupervised. Group counseling is also an option that I did not cover in the chapter. Often, group counseling is facilitated by a licensed professional) and can also be an option.

- Do you feel you have a clear purpose and motivation to do what you need to do in order to live a life you desire and love?

- Do you get to do the things that are important to you?

- Do you suspect that any of the limitations you feel are specifically tied to disability, or is there some other issue/reasoning?

- If you're not currently living a life of things important to you, what would you change in an ideal world?

- Would working with someone help you get clarity and move forward on various fronts in your life? What would you want to work on first?

- Do you have the tools to get what you need?

- Do you have a level of independence and freedom wherever you are to live a life YOU want and desire?

- If you had to make a plan for moving to where you want to be, who would be there? Who and what are you taking with you? What are you leaving behind?

- How do you know it's time for a change?

- I mentioned a number of frustrations and scenarios that occur that can trigger a spiral into depression. Of those, do you share some I've listed? If so, which ones?

- If none of your triggers were listed, what would you say are your triggers?

- What allies can you recruit to help you create change?
- Do you feel like you have something to look forward to that isn't food or the codependency of another person in your life?
- Do you have excitement about fulfilling personal goals and projects? What are you looking forward to in the next three, six or twelve months?
- Do you feel you have genuine friendships that appreciate you and permit you to share candidly and openly without judgment or demeaning how you feel?
- In my book Pack Light: Thoughts for the Journey, I talk about creating a network of folks around you that can be vital to your long-term success. Explore the relevant chapter of that book. I'll talk more about this type of network in the upcoming chapter on Community.
- Whatever you are experiencing, can you name things that you are grateful for? Remember: gratitude is a game changer.

4 / PHYSICAL HEALTH

KEY TAKEAWAYS

- *Having a disability does not give you a pass on the exercise front! In fact, it should be stressed more to us as a way to preserve strength, maintain a healthy weight and fight other diseases.*
- *Physical health is as important for good body image, self-determination and personal confidence as proper hygiene and other forms of self-care. No matter how you look, or how much you fear physical awkwardness, you can be assured when you are doing any type of exercise regimen that you are trying something, and that has got to be a good thing.*
- *All movement is good movement.*
- *Working with a physical therapist can be a good thing, even when you think you are physically unable.*
- *Now more than ever before, there are adaptive physical fitness programs for both adults and*

children, classes and modified equipment available, and this availability is growing each day.

- *It's imperative for parents to realize the crucial role they play in a child's early development and to define their personal outlook on exercise, disability and disease, in addition to how they include their special needs children in chores and other daily activities, especially when they have additional siblings.*

One of the things I wish I hadn't abandoned from childhood is swimming. I absolutely loved to swim! If I had stuck with it, I would've been so much better for it, and likely in much better shape too. I loved the water. There, I had total freedom: the ability to walk and move with zero effort, on my own, buoyed by the weightlessness the water provided. It is likely the reason the doctors say my lungs are in such good shape, and I have yet to experience any respiratory-related illness.

Having a neuromuscular disability, with which the muscles weaken over time - or any other kind of disability diagnosis for that matter - should not be seen as an excuse to completely abandon exercise. I now hate water, but that is only because I've been away from it for so long and I didn't stick with it. For now, unfortunately, my fear of drowning outweighs any physical benefit!

People with disabilities should not be exempt from some form of exercise, even if it's just to move enough through the day to carry out the tasks you need. All movement is good movement.

I'm annoyed at parents who think they will injure and hurt their children if they push them to do things and to try, whatever that looks like. Trust me, it looks awkward and sometimes painful, but it's often not painful to move around. That very push parents can give will mean that muscles can get used just to be used, as opposed to the muscles atrophying, which would mean that the child is the only one who suffers.

This don't-get-hurt mentality is the real culprit behind early death. My Mom pushed me do things, from setting the table and folding the washcloths to wiping down the lower cabinets I could reach from a position on my knees, often scooting around on the floor however I could to get it done. Of course I hated it, but in my twenties, I saw friends who had the same diagnosis as myself unable to make a sandwich or cook anything on top of the stove who later needed their food cut up for them. It was hard to see such a decline in their health over the years, and I know that this was due at least in part to under-utilization of muscles – and, sadly, somewhat responsible for at least one early death. To this day, and even more in our current COVID era, I still cook, I still cut my own food and I'm still able to chew and swallow without assistance. To any advanced person reading this, to anyone who doesn't understand the slow and gradual decline of these motor skills, I realize that these achievements may seem so small to you. They are small... until you can't do them. But now imagine you're a parent of a child with a disability. Consider how your very approach to child rearing, pushing, promoting and encouraging rather than indulgent complacency, giving a pass or permission to do little throughout their day, could mean your child won't be here very long.

I know that what I'm suggesting isn't the be all and end all of saving one's life with a disability. There are things that even exercise can't change: sudden death, for example. It might not make any difference whatsoever. The sad thing with that reality, however, is, that you won't really know what could have been if you're not at least willing to try. Can pushing someone to do more for themselves be to their detriment? I don't think so. Won't a child push back at you when they really can't? Won't you, who sees them daily, be a good judge about when you can push a little more, knowing when your child has reached her or his limit? Of course you will. As much as you care about their wellbeing, you'll recognize the signs of real fatigue and lethargy versus when someone is trying to pull one over on you. Every time, you'll be able to tell the difference between the two.

I'll tell you a secret, and this one is pretty universal among children, disabled or not. Your little one - I know, he or she is so cute, they don't have a manipulative bone in their body, right? Well, I'm going to tell you that the special child you are rearing truly is two different people! They are one person at school and another at home. My parents pushed me at home, but when I got to school, I acted like I couldn't do much of anything.

I remember when my dad didn't want me to have a power chair. They weren't even as sophisticated as they are nowadays, but my first chair was a manual one, and because of the little my dad knew about my disability, he wanted me to try: to push myself for as long as I could. When I got to school, however, a bribe of some candy - a push pop, perhaps - had my peers lining up to push me wherever I needed to go! I relished their help. I didn't have time to be struggling and straining to push myself. Even in elementary school, I was a businesswoman, literally wheeling and dealing (ha-ha!). Collective bargaining, if you will, to get myself to and from my classes. Years later, round about the fourth grade, I got my first power chair and it was on. I was liberated.

In this example, some parents would have let the power chair be their first choice; but, much as my Mom pushed me to do chores on my hands and knees regardless of whether it sounds cruel, my Dad required me to push myself a little longer too: as long as I could. I see that as a good thing.

I know it's a bitter pill to swallow, but you have more control than you think over what happens. The attitude your child develops is a direct response to what YOU say and do for them, throughout their more crucial developmental years.

Caregivers who meet me, and I'm not bragging, will often ask me to talk to this one and that one of their other charges. By that, they are often comparing my abilities to those of their other clients who have similar issues. One even commented: "You can cook? How did you learn to do that?!" And, more bluntly: "My other client, he also has muscular dystrophy, but he can't do half the shit you're doing..." They are home, playing video games, watching television, no desire to further their education, get a job or even see if there is one out there to be had that they can in fact do (there are, by the way: they may be hard to find, but in truth it's more about attitudinal barriers than about one's capability.)

I want to be clear: I'm not overlooking the serious effects of any neuromuscular disease. That is not it at all. And you may think I'm being tough on parents of children with disabilities, but when a parent brings an eighteen-year-old to your office saying here, do something, fix him, you see the error of a parent's way. Such was the case when a mother brought her six-foot-tall son to my office one day. Ms. Tracee, Ms. Tracee, she said, he so messy, he don't clean up, he eat everything...

My message to all parents of children with disabilities is: This young man was fully physically able to clean up for himself and after himself. He had Autism. The simple fact was that, at age 18, the mother wanted me to assist the child. Think about it. This meant that for 18 years, she hadn't once taken the time to help him learn how to best care for himself and manage his own self-care needs. He was able to get a job. In fact, he always had a job, ever since I started working with him. What often happened is that he lost interest, grew bored and quit the jobs he obtained.

No, you can't blame the parents for everything, but no one taught this young man about money, about a paycheck to pay for things, about taking care of his home, his room, vacuuming... These were all things he could provably do in the home, because he was often tasked with these same kind of chores at the work environments where he would easily get a job.

But NO ONE took the time. Instead, they gave him a pass, as many parents and even those in society will do. You know what society is already saying:

Why work out?

Why go out?

Why not just collect a government check?

Why aren't you receiving disability checks?

How much is your disability check?

You work?

Outside the home?

Why?

How?

For what?

What happens when the parents dies?

What happens when the Aunt can't put up with her disabled niece or nephew because he lacks basic skills? What happens when we require nothing of people with disabilities? What happens is that nursing facilities fill up with just as many 40-something's with disabilities as those who are supposed to be living there at 70-90.

We could mitigate this housing crisis, this need for care

crisis, by doing whatever we can at the beginning, and not simply bringing folks to service providers to fix everything at the end. What the mother asked me to do wasn't something that could be fixed between the ages of 18 and 40. I could do something to help, and slowly we worked on a few things. At this point, though, he's disinterested and doesn't see the benefit, when his parents have made life so easy up until now. What needed to occur really needed to happen from ages 0 to 18.

My parents never acted like I had a disability. They made some concessions, of course, but they expected the same things from me as they did from my brother - although I still feel like I got away with a lot by virtue of being female. My parents realized things might have taken a little longer, it might not have been perfect, it was going to be my version; but the point was always going to be that I tried, and they had the patience to let me do it, however long it took, and NOT rushing to my aid at the least bit of adversity. Their attitude gave me the where-withal to finish, which ultimately built sufficient confidence to see things through and to do the best I could. Too often, parents rush in to fix things, to ease the path and to remove all thorns. These thorns, however, are important for life: to get prickled a bit, to hit brick walls, to fall down, but eventually, with guid-ance, patience and support, to course-correct and find a new way.

Even at times when I tell my mom, I really do have a disability, she says 'Where?" Looking at me expectantly as if it should pop up from my wheelchair.

Of course, there is so much I can't do physically, but all that work I was doing even at four and five years old on tasks that seemed so small - and were to every able-bodied person who hasn't seen a person with a disability struggle - still keep my muscles going all these years later.

What's more, doing stuff makes a child feel included. Their siblings won't later resent them for not trying, for getting the pass. Furthermore, as much as you'd hate for your other children to have to take care of your child with special needs once you die, this can-do attitude and push might often help provide at least some assurance that later in life, they too will become the champion you once were for their siblings' rights, safety and access to inclusion. With luck, they will go on helping them live in the community and be there for them after you are gone. Seeing them try offers an opportunity for mutual respect. Even children can tell when everyone is bending over backwards to accommodate this one person, but your approach to everything will give them cues on what to do now, not to mention later when, at some point, they will be in charge.

Physical activity, doing what you can, means so much. Start early to find whatever it is that can be done. Get out of your comfort zone to see what other parents are doing. What does the physical and occupational therapist say?

Finally, we have to examine why we're so resistant to the push for kids to do some physical activity. Yes, you don't want them to hurt, but is there possibly guilt somewhere? Why? You didn't cause their disability. *You are not responsible that it occurred, however you feel about that.* Don't let guilt be a pass for inaction. Assumptions, doctor's prognoses and your own personal dismal outlook about disability must be challenged and confronted. You must let go of your own personal guilt about your current state, and as a parent, you must let go of parental guilt that does nothing for anyone. This is your child to lead and his/her very first example of how to handle their disability. Their ultimate success and a bright future starts with you.

TAKE ACTION ON PHYSICAL HEALTH

- While I have touted the benefits of activity when you have a muscle disease or neurological problem, **exercise is not always the best course of action.** There are other forms of movement and breathing that also constitute exercise. Think about breathing, about yoga, even typing on a computer! Meditation and stretching can be low-impact forms of exercise, too.
- Overexerting yourself may have devastating and ill-advised effects on your stamina, cause increased fatigue and just be a bad idea overall, but that's not to say that you can't move around, even if you're a wheelchair user. I say again: any kind of movement is a good idea, no matter what.
- As early as I can remember, Richard Simmons was one of the first fitness gurus that I saw coming on the scene with a seated workout. He did everything from a chair, surrounded by people with disabilities of varying ability levels all doing a version of

whatever they could. This very video is now free on YouTube.

- Remember that physical health isn't just exercise and eating healthy. There's something to be said for brain exercises, and even for the little movements of scooting yourself around in your chair or preparing a simple meal. As a writer, I often wondered if typing burned any calories, and I was pleasantly surprised to learn that according to Harvard Health Publications, typing on a computer burns 41 calories per half hour for a 125-pound person. (A 155-pound person burns 51 calories typing for 30 minutes and a 185-pound person burns 61 calories doing the same job.) This was quite a revelation for me, and I now realize that everything counts, so don't knock it until you try it! This isn't much but it was still quite cool. I burned a lot of calories typing this book, by the way.

- Brain games, the ones that became popular during the pandemic of 2020, can also be forms of engagement and, yes, exercise.

- As trainers continue to find their niches, there are a number of trainers that specialize in assisting people with disabilities. Most offer one-time consultations, and you can arrange to find a series of exercises and a regimen that's best for you, while being assured that they will be considerate of your abilities and needs.

- Gyms are also becoming more and more open, with some even shutting down their normal operating hours to offer a few hours that will be dedicated to people with disabilities. Many have volunteers and certified trainers leading programs so that we can feel more comfortable working out, even providing one-on-one assistance to help you complete your workout. To find these types of programs, ask your local Center for Independent Living and the local Rehabilitation Centers, as well as physical and occupational therapists, about resources in your community. Also, don't be afraid to start these kinds of groups yourself where you see a need. Look specifically for the keywords and tags "adaptive fitness" and "adaptive training".

• If there was a physical activity you did as a child or adolescent, never stop finding a way to do that. Don't let age, stigma or the sometimes-weakening progression of your disease keep you from that thing, nor surgeries or bouts of illness. Try to ALWAYS return to that one thing or some modification of it, even if you could once do it solo but can't anymore: there are supports out there, actual medical equipment, that could make it easier or more accessible.

5 / TRANSPORTATION

KEY TAKEAWAYS

- Transportation is such a vital key to a mobile society. It makes everything work, and when there is no adequate system available, whether public or private, this can mean life and death.
- We should be afforded equal opportunity to pursue all types of driving options, and the technology supports exist for us as people with disabilities. However, we should be the first not to take this endeavor lightly, whether you can pursue it with some of the most advanced technology or the tech isn't there for your situation just yet. If it's easy or complicated (and expensive), more than just a personal desire and physical capability should be considered when making such a weighty decision.
- Don't ever let case managers, family, or others who can't fathom the types of advancements they haven't seen with their own eyes underestimate

what kinds of technology is available and undermine your research.

- Your inability (and your unwillingness -if that's the case) to drive should not be a factor when considering whether you've attained a certain level of success. There are numerous other ways to reach your destinations and your goals without the operation of your vehicle.
- Whatever you do, keep an open mind and think outside the box for new ways to reach this and every single goal you've set for yourself.

It seemed some of my worst, most notorious bullies would always take the form of bus drivers. Not sure what it was about me, or whether it was even about me at all, but I just could not catch a break with the folks tasked to drive me somewhere, whether that was to all my schooling, K-12, or even later when I would start going back and forth to college following gradua-tion. That little short bus that pulled up often had just the angriest driver, often a woman, who had to rise from the sweaty leather throne she'd been sitting in all day, climb from the bus and walk around to operate the lift and strap my wheelchair in once inside. Such drivers would never greet me with a kind word but a full-on nasty attitude. I never did understand the reason behind it: only that it was a most unpleasant experience for most of my life. In elementary school, back when people with disabilities were still being bussed to schools that were not located in their own neighborhoods, I had such a long ride to school that as soon as I got on the bus they seemed to start in on me about falling asleep. I mean, what else was I supposed to do for an almost hour-long ride picking up other children and staring at the back of the driver's balding, graying head?

This mean-ass bus driver situation followed me into adulthood. While I now understand that it wasn't about me at all, perhaps it was rather just a strong propelling hand to make me hate being at the mercy of someone else, thus giving me a strong sense of desire to either make enough money to be chauffeured around like a bigwig (I wish), or at least pray that the technology was developed for me to drive my own vehicle.

Thank God those types of systems *were* developed... kinda. When I was researching options to see how in the world I could possibly drive my own car, the Department of Rehabilitation Services, or DRS (now called The Department for Aging and Rehabilitation Services, or DARS) would be an organization that helped me tremendously. But it wasn't easy by any means.

First, I had an assessment at their Rehabilitation Center in another part of Virginia. I can't name names here, but it was about a three-hour drive from where I lived. It was a nice small town, but there was a weird feeling about it for me as a person with a disability. I looked it up on the Internet, probably before Yelp was even invented, and after reading some of things I uncovered, I decided I just could not stay there overnight. For the record, the place has a bit of a reputation for police being called often, and for unruly young people.

What annoyed me is that not only is the Center a place for people with disabilities to learn, have assessments and rehabilitate, I later found that it's also used for kids with behavioral issues, as well as some violent offenders involved with drugs and other substance abuse who also happen to be people with disabilities.

I'm not even sure how I was able to get my evaluation done in one day. If I'm being honest, I probably used my disability in some fashion and my advocacy skills in another. The agency was only going to pay so much for this assessment. Side note: remember that in every endeavor of yours as a person with a disability, a minority or just about anything that makes you look different, a case manager somewhere is making his or her own determination about your abilities, whether well-intentioned or ignorant. Often, they do this having not a single accurate fact about you as a person, or about your capabilities; yet they'll make sometimes devastating decisions about what you can and cannot do – and, worse, what they will and will not fund.

This is unfair. Such is life. Well-meaning people will make assumptions about your disability, and they in their all-too-powerful positions will make decisions that deny you the very right to live and thrive. This sounds dramatic, I realize that. But imagine being denied the right to have an assessment: zero funds to float that assessment, being left to figure it out on my own and out of pocket. Imagine their 'yes' being the only thing between me and my driving freedom. Again, yes, that sounds a little dramatic, but when you realize that transportation gets you to the job, the job provides the healthcare, the job provides the money so you can live and pay for the housing, the quality of life, the access to social opportunities, leisure and recreation, to the doctor's office for regular check-ups or even to the emergency room? If I were a parent myself, or if I had to help my own aging mother, of if I needed to get myself to the emergency room… and on and on… Does this still seem overly dramatic to you?

I probably told them it would be cheaper for me to go down for the day, rather than them having to pay for an aide to accompany me.

I felt like my Dad might have felt when he advocated for me in elementary school. I think of him as I write this very piece. Who knew if what I asked was going to work? - but let's just try it, anyway.

While I was able to go down and get my driving evaluation done in one day, the news wasn't good.

The pull-and-push hand controls they tested me on wouldn't work. With my left hand, I had to pull the lever back to stop the vehicle and push it forward to accelerate. With my right hand, I had to operate the steering wheel. I clearly remember going down a dirt hill and getting stuck, with the therapist right there beside me. I couldn't push the lever forward far enough with my left hand to get us back up the hill.

It was easy to blame them. Who in the hell has a hill for your first driving simulation?! The truth was, though, the system was too hard for me. I didn't have the upper body strength to do that, and thus the evaluation was over.

Despite it all, I actually had a nice driver for once. She took me to McDonald's and, after eating, I slept the rest of the way home, feeling defeated.

I really thought that was it: that my driving dreams had been quashed and that I was doomed to a future populated by hellish bus drivers... until the counselor mentioned a therapist who had more extensive equipment.

When I met him, I was in awe. He was a therapist, and he was so good looking that my first thought was: *there is no way I'm going to pass this - how will I ever concentrate with him sitting right beside me giving me instructions?!* I had visions of driving us into a tree as a result, getting flashes of inspiration for a potential future book title: *How I Killed My Fine-Ass Driving Instructor: A Post-Mortem Memoir.*

In truth, I did have a hard time driving with him initially, but the controls were out of sight. For the first few attempts, my right hand was on the joystick that controlled everything from the accelerator to the brake, just like driving my wheelchair. The steering wheel was spinning around untouched, like Drew Barrymore in *The Exorcist*.

Unfortunately, I would jerk the vehicle (and my fine ass instructor, to my dismay) stopping and starting around and around the parking lot until we both had a headache. This van had the absolute most extensive (and expensive) hand controls. I hadn't seen anything like it. The joystick operated almost the entire driving system. On the left were a series of buttons where you changed gears by pressing corresponding buttons, as well as turning things on and off: the lights, turn signals, wipers, horn and all the rest, simply by pressing a button. It was amazing. Up close and personal, really getting to see the vehicle and how it operated, brought everything to life.

It was easy. All I had to do was build my confidence, because after all it was also several tons of machinery that in the event of an accident could injure both others and myself, fatally. There's that little word with really horrifying consequences: another reason why I couldn't take what I was embarking on so lightly. This was probably the harder thing to grapple with as a new driver: perhaps even one that could be usefully added to the physical and mental driving assessments required before driving such an extensive system. Then again, maybe it shouldn't, simply because they don't do it for the many non-disabled sixteen-year-old kids who have only to pass a few tests and are granted the right to drive. We certainly don't need any more barriers than there already are. I know, because I confronted them all.

Still, the fact remains that there is no mention of testing your acuity, let alone moral obligations, for when you're driving such an expensive, altered piece of machinery. Nowhere is it discussed what an accident can do to a disabled driver mentally and physically. Yes, these things happen to non-disabled people all the time too, but imagine being in such an accident when you are already disabled. Talk about a double whammy.

Finally, something I never had any idea about but wish I had known is the astronomical cost of maintenance for a modified vehicle. When you boil it down, it's like you're maintaining two separate vehicles. I talked about this in the health section, that maintaining my body seemed to require not just my own team of folks for normal human physiology, but another team for the disabled part of me. It seemed the same for my vehicle. There are frequent system issues which must be seen to by an electrical specialist, the closest of which to me was located in Maryland, about a 90 minute drive for my home. Then there are your regular car maintenance people, the Jiffy Lubes and the Merchants of this world, who covered and fixed only the mechanical aspects of the car as a regular vehicle. For perspective, the modifications alone at my time of purchase were around $45K, and that was on top of the sticker price of the vehicle, a Chrysler Dodge Grand Caravan, which, with the ramp already installed, would run from a mere $35K (if you're lucky) to more like $55K. Yes, fifty-five thousand dollars.

Secondly, I would learn that I could not modify a vehicle with more than 12,000 miles on it, because it couldn't have any preexisting conditions. I bought my vehicle about just that, it was a year old and it had approximately 10K miles on it. The reason for this is that you don't want the vehicle to age out of the modifications. They should age together, or you won't get the full use out of it.

Another expense is that of hiring an instructor. The therapist I had to teach me driving was using his own vehicle, with the modifications I was going to be using, and it cost me about $20K.

This of course included his time, education and expertise, but also his travel, gas, hotel stay, meals and other per diem expenses. He would stay in the area not far from where I lived for almost two whole weeks and we went out everyday, practicing using the specially adapted van. Over the course of that two weeks, I would rack up over 40 hours of hands-on driving, in parking lots and other areas where there weren't many cars around, until he thought I was ready to venture out on the main roads and highways with everyone else. The number of practice hours will vary but are roughly the same for almost everyone. You can either do it in the timeframe your PT/Driving Instructor therapist is there, or you can't. As we neared the end of his stay, I finally started to improve. The headache-inducing jerky movements ceased and soon I was on Route 66 with the rest of them, gunning a happy 45 in the slow lane. Yeah Baby. Check out your girl!

I used his vehicle to do the driving test and that first time, I got one little restriction: highway. It sounded big; it wasn't. I just drove on it anyway. If a police officer asked, I was practicing. Luckily this and some of the vehicle modifications were paid for by the state rehabilitation agency. This isn't something I'll just go back for once my current vehicle bites the dust. This will likely, back then, have been a one-time thing for me and every other person at that time who was able to get that service. Unfortunately, with budget cuts and spending limits, I know there are currently tighter restrictions on what state vocational rehabilitation centers are going to pay. That means if this is something you strongly desire, you will incur these costs out of pocket. At the time I learned to drive, however, there weren't the number of crowd-sourced programs that are available today. With the creation of such platforms as GoFundMe, you have a chance to raise the funds for your independence: a chance unheard of in the early 2000s, when I was doing what I needed.

When you look at all the cost details I've outlined here, you realize we're now talking about an effort that costs almost 100K, including the vehicle, the modifications, the driving assessments, the therapist - and all for a vehicle that will last you maybe fifteen years if you really take care of it. Considering the likelihood of the equipment/modifications aging well, I can tell you that this timeline is not guaranteed. The maintenance is something to think about continuously. Those costs will only increase, as maintenance visits become more frequent and as the vehicle ages, sinking dollar after dollar into it.

You have to be real and you have to swallow a pill that begs the question: can I physically do this? Can I fiscally do this? Can I mentally do this? If I can't, what is the alternative? Being realistic, can I afford this or would a nice house or condo in the city be just fine with me? This is the price you pay for your independence, of course, but if I had to play the other side of the coin? Honestly, with all that money, you could have a nice down payment on a condo in Arlington, Virginia, or any urban area when transit options are more plentiful. As devastating as not having the freedom to drive seemed to me, people make it in life without a personally-owned vehicle every single day, and you will too.

However, if the technology exists and all other factors are in place, shouldn't you at least try? Will you know what you could have accomplished if you didn't even try?

I persevered despite my case manager asking me about my health and almost deterring me by saying, inaccurately, that due to my health condition they shouldn't support me. Such experiences can certainly cause you to question your own health and abilities, but it's essential to move forward no matter what and in spite of whatever others think about your capabilities. *He might get hit by a bus,* this is what I often thought; *should he not eat lunch?*

The car could be totaled through no fault of your own, your health could fail, you could hit someone, someone could hit you... but what's important is that these things could happen regardless of disability. As such, whether or not you're approved, find a way to the things you want: the freedoms you want out of life. If you aren't approved, simply go around those folks to find someone to help you make it happen.

My own parents had plenty of advanced technology throughout our house, from a lift that deploys from the ceiling (barrier free lift) to a power chair: as I mentioned, I got my first version of a power chair in elementary school. As for driving, they weren't home when I was working with the instructor so they didn't really get to see the vehicle and understand its capabilities until the company that completed the modifications drove it to our house for me. Meanwhile, they saw it as 'just this thing I was working on' while they and many others wondered how in the world it was even possible. How will it be when Stevie Wonder, or any blind person for that matter, takes their first trip to a gig in an autonomous vehicle, also known as a self-driving car? I can tell you: it will be completely crazy! Innovative and amazing. Technology continues to advance, giving us hope for a normal life and a level playing field to create that life.

Driving is liberating. When I'm in my van, out there with everyone else, music blasting with a lot of bass, there is no other feeling quite like it. It's a feeling of normalcy, of being like everyone else. Yes, there will come a time when I can no longer drive, when muscles, cognitive function or who knows what may well throw a spanner in the works; but right now, you and

I both have what we need. If you can, if there is even a slight possibility of you getting to your goal, you should exhaust all options.

The reason for going into detail here about all the costs is that I haven't read a single book that's given me the tools to make an informed decision, or an awareness of exactly what I would have to go through to understand all that's involved. In short, no book I read outlined the ways in which I as a Black woman with a disability would be discriminated against.

A part of the story I left off is that when I first moved to the county I was in, I was denied paratransit service. Paratransit is the door-to-door service that picks up people with disabilities from their homes. Usually you have to arrange your ride 24 hours in advance for a ride the following day, and then only if a slot is available. When I scheduled my first ride, the driver looked at me and refused. I had to take it higher. Ultimately, the owner came to my house and told me and my dad that I was too heavy for the lift: that the lift would fail. At this point I was in my twenties, after riding a school bus for my entire life, after being in an adjacent county riding their Paratransit for years, before moving to Ass-Backwards-Ville. They also suggested they weigh me in the bus, take me off the bus, then weight it again to see what the difference was. We could have sued them; we should have. Instead, I went to a special rehabilitation place that weighed me and my chair, supplying the company with the official weight that finally permitted me to ride.

The level of absurdity should be appalling to you. It was to me. In the moment, the full weight - pun not intended - of what they were doing should have been clearer to me.

Looking back on it now, I cannot believe the audacity of yet more people in positions of power, denying even basic access to services for community residents such as myself. Transportation has such a freeing capacity that everyone should have and that everyone needs, whatever form it's in. Everyone has a need for it. It means access to medical care, to competitive and gainful employment, to recreation, fun and entertainment. Without it, it's possible to fall into isolation, depression, even death in the event of an emergency. It is a vital component in the life of a person with a disability.

Sadly, there are so many more horror stories: some outlined, some never told. While I realize just how much of a push this gave me overall, no one should have go through that. Ultimately, it was another bullet point on my already extensive list of why driving would become such a burning desire of mine. I could not give up: the technology was there, the funds were made available, the powers that be eventually got in line, and it was up to me to grab the opportunity that was looming in the not too distant future. You will have to find a way to make it happen, and trust me, you can.

TAKE ACTION ON TRANSPORTATION

- Before even thinking about driving, I don't care what disability you have: *there may be a way*. It might not be easy – I know your *life* as a person with a disability is not easy. It might cost much more - money can be raised. Some may not grasp the technology that's available or that is developing all the time, even in the time that has lapsed since my penning these words. Finally, bear in mind that what you need and want to do might not always look like you envisioned, but that doesn't mean it can't still be some form of independence that gets you what you need. You must first keep an open mind about technological advances you have yet to encounter. Just because you haven't seen something yet does not mean it doesn't exist, or that people aren't actively working on solutions for the very problems you have at this very moment. I mean, just think: right now, we know that someone is out there perfecting the autonomous car, poised to release it just as soon as they iron out one more issue (um, that would be avoiding collisions with pedestrians... I mean, that is a big deal.) My point is that look how far technology has come! Look how quickly a vaccine can be created with the whole world working on it together. Bottom line: the research to solve complex problems does not ever stop. I looked at the equipment updates for my vehicle just the other day: that has improved even in the ten-plus years that I've been driving.

- Find ways to challenge your readiness and build confidence. Be like your nondisabled peers who never think about injury to anyone. They just think, *this is what I want, I can do it.* Never mind what scientists say about the brain and maturity, and that most boys especially should wait until they are older to drive. Absolutely no one buys into this, though: at fifteen and sixteen, it's just our cultural norm that this is the age to drive. People with disabilities are often stuck waiting on technology and permissions to coincide before moving forward. Ain't nobody got time for that. Let's go!

- I keep waiting for corporate outside-the-box thinking to occur with transportation. Until it does, you have to think outside the box yourself for getting around town and country. Sadly, as advanced as we are, there is no plane that I've seen - unless Elon Musk is hiding something in space - that will permit a wheelchair user to remain in their chair for travel. You do realize this is doable? The hold-up is the airlines' monetary hit from removing two seats. Wheelchairs are crash-tested, by the way. What we're waiting for is someone to green-light this as a worthy endeavor, declaring that they should be accessible as a company. Until then, you *can* still travel by plane, even if you need help transferring. There are people to help you transfer into an aisle chair, to transfer you again to a plane seat, and to "properly" store your wheelchair in the cargo area of the plane to help you get on with your life. Might it sustain damage? Of course, but you have recourse for damages. It's not easy, no, but it's worth it.

- Hiring a driver: sometimes it might be a good option. You never know who you'll find. I mean, what if someone worked for a commercial vehicle company and didn't mind driving you daily at a set time for your job, recurring appointment or just about anything? This is doable. The hard part is knowing where to post this kind of need.

- Someone going the same way you are - a coworker or someone working in the vicinity of your place of employment/business. In a forthcoming book, tentatively titled *Side Hustle School for Those with Chronic Conditions*, I'll be talking about this again, and more in depth.

- Your peers may be an option for transportation assistance. College and of-age school friends as well as retired seniors are still quite capable of driving, despite the ageism issues they face.

- While not immediate and while you may be tired of all the advocacy that must occur in every facet of life – see? Told ya! It never ends! - you have to know that transportation or some kind of community effort is doable. In many smaller and rural areas, folks have banded together to find a ride and their effort has grown to become the type of transit system that just works: tailored to those populations' needs. In fact, this is how many a larger, robust transit system starts: with one vehicle, with one volunteer, with one driver, all with a mission to get folks where they need to go. Start small, with just one bus, one driver, one mechanic that knows how to fix the special parts of vehicle AND the lift issues that arise.

- Find the funds. If you have them, great! If not, you can do some grassroots organizing. Find folks to help you. Sometimes living in a smaller area can be a good thing. The local folks who've lived there for a time can see you trying. They've known you your entire life and buy in to the story of your *why*. It's the human interest portion of the late-night news segment, and this one and that one rally support to make it happen. It might look like someone down the road at the largest dealer in the town gifting you – well, maybe steeply discounting - your first ramp van. When called upon, the community can rally behind you, but you have to be open to outside the box thinking, with humility and a willing disposition to try new things to get on the path toward what you want. Anything can happen and you never, ever know.

- What can be your motivation? What will propel you to meet a "no" and move forward to the next step? For me, it took almost ten years of denials, setbacks and several firm no's to realize my dream. Not everyone can stick to that and still believe it's

something they will attain. What will keep you
motivated as you move forward through life? Read
this final story of a vision of what can be, to
motivate you. Also, check out resources and articles
on the blog about transportation resources.

A final story of motivation for helping me see that I could do
this: a friend of mine had a similar form of Muscular Dystrophy, and we used to be the best of friends. He was a white guy,
and he actually drove by my house. I can't remember if he
called me and said 'hey, come outside' or exactly how that
occurred, but there I was, at the end of my driveway, watching
him in this white van, driving from his wheelchair, the
instructor beside him in the passenger seat. I'll never forget the
smile on his face as he stopped to chat for what seemed like the
briefest of moments before he was off, driving to the end of the
road, where I stared after him, in an almost euphoric state. He
might as well have been riding off into the big blue skyline, for
how dazed and confused I was after he drove off. Why, we rode
the short yellow bus together! Interestingly, he hadn't ever been
by my house to visit me before: probably because he couldn't
yet drive. In any case, I believe that the single stop he made to
come by my home that day was God's way of showing me what
was possible. That it was doable, that he had done it, and that if
I tried hard enough and was serious, I could do it too. As you
grow up, you have to use these things not for resentment, envy
and jealousy. I personally plead the fifth on what emotions ran
through me at the time – to be honest, it felt like he was rubbing
it in, although I doubt that's what it was - but thinking back on
it now, I know he was just there to tell me, to demonstrate for
me that I too could do this. Here he was doing it: that could be
me! That WOULD be me! Eventually. I was so excited. I had

so many questions, I wanted to see more of the controls he was using, I wanted a ride in that damn van!!! "Let me in!" I thought excitedly.

I didn't know my route would be so difficult with the discrimination I encountered. My case manager at the time denied me almost five times before my dad came to help advocate on my behalf yet again. Dad sat in on one of the meetings with my case manager. Finally, I decided it was time for me to get off the rejection train: leaving behind the inexplicable denials over four or five years of my life, getting another case manager who miraculously got the funding support for the modifications approved with his first attempt. He was either so new they approved it, or it was because they'd seen my name come through for the umpteenth time. What is so odd but funny is that this particular Rehabilitation office gave me an award almost a year later to show off my "new van". All the case managers came out to the parking lot to see me operate it. I started the vehicle up and showed them all the hand controls and the steering wheel turning on its own, to their amazement and my own internal glee.

To start all that in motion, I needed my friend to plant the seeds of driving for myself one day, whatever his motives were. I needed the rub of the initial denial from the Paratransit company; I needed the mean bus drivers and every other single adversity to get on my last nerve and motivate me through this process. I needed to understand that when you hit roadblocks, you have options: that operating the pull and push lever with the left hand and the steering wheel in the right hand might not have worked, but that even more advanced technology could be had. You cannot always see all the options there at once, but you have to keep pushing past each barrier to find the next option.

6 / HOUSING

KEY TAKEAWAYS

- Housing issues, as much as if not more than the current health care disparities and crisis is and will continue to be our next crisis among people with disabilities, young families with disabled children and the elderly.
- Complex housing issues are being solved in small pockets and we will need to develop an approach that can be replicated throughout the United States and beyond.
- Everyone can be more open and think outside the box for shared living opportunities that can be a win-win for all involved
- Youth, young adults with Intellectual and Developmental Disabilities, adults with physical disabilities and the homeless could become the most displaced populations without a solid plans to

house and address the housing needs of these groups
- There is no right or wrong housing model to strive for, it's whatever works for the people involved who need safe housing
- What you had in mind for your living arrangements may not look like the vision you hold right now, it's important to not only make peace so long as you are able to have choice and feel safe, and that is okay.

"There's a real crisis," said Shawn Ullman, senior director for national initiatives at The Arc. *"People are having to get creative. The old way of doing things is not sustainable. A lack of safe and affordable housing is the number one issue for adults with intellectual and developmental disabilities."*

The only thing left out of that statement is that many people assume that people with only ("only") physical disabilities do not face the same dire housing challenges as people with ID and DD, which is not at all the case.

Now, you may just live under a rock, or maybe you know zero people with disabilities anywhere in the US, if you don't yet realize that we're in a housing crisis and have been for some time. But whatever you do or don't know, the fact is that safe and stable housing is one of the most important things in life, yet it's also affected by so many different factors: the economy, jobs, government, climate, public transit, accessibility, housing inventory levels and more. All of these factors make affordability and accessibility in housing such a volatile subject.

Sadly, affordable housing isn't an issue unique to people

with disabilities – but, on the bright side, that fact can actually help us in our advocacy for more of it. Because so many people need to be able to live and work in their neighborhoods, housing inventory must be more affordable. For people with disabilities, there must also be accessibility - but when you have the audacity to try and combine this request with affordability, you come across a bit of an oddity: more often than not, the two don't coexist. If you're fortunate enough to find something affordable, the modifications and upgrades would be too costly. Conversely, when the home is built to be fully accessible, such modifications and upgrades built into the home make the price tag insurmountable.

For a time, many were on board with universal design in housing, making more homes that feature accessible components, even offering retrofitting that, with some finagling, could make a new construction more accessible. The problem with the UD movement was the fact that accessibility was still relative, and as such did not always fit individual users. It was more of a blanket way of "fixing" the problem – and, as we know all too well, disability is often just too individualized for one size to fit all. For most people with disabilities, the fact remains that rigging up and fixing things to fit you to the fullest extent possible is what we do. We simply adapt.

The other big issue beyond accessibility and affordability - which will likely be a mainstay for some time - is one simple question: *For us, what and where is home, and who defines that?*

Solving housing issues in my profession was always a losing battle. This has always been an especially difficult task where I lived, as well as many other suburban and rural areas. The inventory is low; you have be dirt poor to get some type of subsidy; and while there may exist a single unit that meets your needs, it's full. You're basically waiting for folks to die so that your name can move up the wait list and you can get that long-awaited call. What's more, even if you get that call some day, it will have gone out to hundreds, sometimes thousands, on the wait list. Even then, ONLY the person that has the down payment ready, clears the credit and background checks, is ready to move that instant, and of course has the good fortune to actually pick up that one fateful call will finally get the golden ticket.

For us to get ready, it just takes a little more of everything. What's more, those who make the housing rules and regulations don't often take into account an added room for live-in caregivers, a little additional room for the extra equipment we may need for everyday living, and numerous other things that can make the home downright uninhabitable if you have a disability.

Such restrictions further impede people with disabilities, making institutions and multi-person housing the only realistic options. Yes, sometimes we get support: federally mandated support through the Centers for Medicaid and Medicare Services, and Long Term Care support programs through the health insurance. So what's the problem? Well, such support was never meant to be 24 hours. If you need 24-hour support, well sorry: according to government officials, it's time for you to go into a nursing facility. Directing your own care and the people caring for you just isn't enough if you become sick. If you require a temporary stay in the hospital, and maybe later rehabilitation, the services for your in-home care aren't designed to pause. You either have them or you don't, and when you leave your home, you pretty much kiss those services goodbye.

This sounds devastating, and it is. It might sound even a bit exaggerated to you; but the stories of this happening are real and well-documented. I've seen cases where the family of an elderly person has sold the home, or let it go into foreclosure, without telling the family member. In other cases, we managed to get someone a certain number of hours for care - say 16 hours during the day and partly into the night – but the family actually refused the help that would cost them no money out of pocket: help tat would clear the way for the patient to move back home. Such family members often cited work, children, reluctance to render care, or other obligations prohibiting them for providing care. (Never mind the fact that with 16 hours of care, there were only another 8 hours left to be covered - which, with strategic arrangements, should have been spent sleeping.) Even with such a set up, it was still just too burdensome. The funds existed, yet the heart to ease the move back to the disabled person's comfortable home, where they could begin to make improvements in their health and eventually thrive, just wasn't enough of a reason for their family to make it happen. The person in question was elderly, but this does not happen just to elderly people: middle aged folks, even young folks, as well as Veterans home from war, can ultimately face this kind of plight. They remain in the nursing facility despite being capable of thriving at home until they die, their death often accelerated by the lack of options and the frustration of knowing that, given the chance, they could be successful.

What's wrong with the nursing facility? Well, there are some good ones - few, but some. But said facilities would be exponentially better if they paid staff an appropriate wage, promoted better training standards and enforced health, sanitary and safety standards. Nothing unveiled and illuminated the state of play in nursing homes better than COVID-19. Talk about a blinding beam of light in the darkness. COVID-19 shone a light on things many of us already knew were happening in both public and privately-run facilities. To put it like Whoopi Goldberg in Ghosts: "Molly, you in danger, girl." And if I may put my own spin on this famous statement: "Molly, you in danger girl...of dying!"

Secondly, in the scheme of things, if we find housing within our means, we end up unable to pay for the additional support required. There's no money left over for a caregiver to come in, out of pocket. If you have a Medicaid standard issue assistance, it only pays a fraction of the care hours needed: never a living wage, and barely minimum wage. And forget it if you are on public benefits, such as social security disability income. These limits make it impossible for a home of your own to be realized.

With that said, some creative, out-of-the box housing options that people have managed to put together have actually worked. I'll cover some of the innovative ways that it could end up working for you.

First, some parents of disabled youth have pooled their resources with other parents to purchase a townhome or condo and create a roommate situation for their son or daughter who has special needs, paired with another family that also has a son or daughter with special needs - usually two of the same gender. Some such parents also go on to hire a college student of a similar age to their own children, or a behavioral support person (a growing career sector) - or even a general, unskilled caregiver - to live in or at least check in regularly to ensure that everyone has what they need and is safe. Once a week, this support person may shop for groceries and other household necessities, ensure bills are paid, check safety issues, and communicate about any other needs or concerns. The support person can then report directly to the parents/guardians, even if they don't live nearby, and can also provide activities for the tenants to do if the youth don't already hold some sort of employment.

Similarly, parents are also creating group home situations where two or more caregivers hired for that particular home can provide care for up to four residents, each having varying levels of friendship with each other and their own autonomous outside activities, such as employment or recreation. A similar set-up to the roommate situation - however, some multi-group and shared living settings require 501c3 status, with separate banking accounts and a Board of Directors, for what is ultimately a nonprofit organization. That way, any potential income is pooled into the nonprofit in order to maintain the property with the site's income, rather than billing individuals. These more complex arrangements do require lawyers and accountants and official paperwork filing, but as such are still completely doable.

Some of these set-ups give youth the feeling of living on their own, providing the experience of what it's really like and helping them to cultivate options for what to do in the event that parents die or become ill. There can be a number of detailed written instructions and directives set forth. Best of all, the youth will already have some confidence about influencing their own lives, increasing their independence and self-reliance.

One of the main goals with these kinds of arrangements relates to the long-term friendships that are formed, reflecting the youths' ability to get along with different and diverse groups of people, some of whom ultimately provide their care. A second plus is simply financial: the joint setup means that no one family is taxed more heavily than the others. However, solid legal agreements - especially about home ownership, division of labor, dissolution and/or eviction - will be a must: one of the ultimate keys to any family's long term success in such a situation. Finally, the person with a disability can feel a sense of empowerment and connection to folks outside their family, which is one of the hardest parts of developing independence. Growing out of that initial dependency is difficult, as youth learn to trust others beyond their parents and guardians. To be frank, another hidden benefit is that setting this up promptly can alleviate both the burden and the ensuing resentment a sibling might have, making them a little more willing to offer support and direct these processes if all they have to do is tweak the arrangement rather than setting it all up from scratch. Siblings, as future caretakers in the parent's untimely death or illness, are never guaranteed. While that can be sad, it's the reality.

As more aging children with disabilities remain with their families in the family home, most parents fail to realize how important friendships can be for quality of life in the long term. A chief complaint from parents of children with special needs is the lack of friendships and engagement available to their child, especially as they age. Not only do programs dry up after a certain age, this can be a self-fulfilling prophecy if the child is not strongly encouraged to be social, or at least gain some level of social skill to get along with others. Unfortunately, this issue only seems to worsen as the child ages.

Some of these cooperative set-ups provide built-in buddies for youth in the home and are thus a surefire way to promote friendship and engagement. This is similar to the time-honored strategy of older widows who find community and reduce loneliness and isolation by creating communities and, yes, moving in, together.

As I think about my own housing situation and those of other people with physical disabilities, especially with mobility issues, I also have had to think about my own limits. What were the options going to be for me? As a planner and thinker, I had thoroughly developed and even begun to realize two possible contingency plans, while also realizing that even the best laid plans can go asunder.

I have created two robust options that I have presented to families as possible solutions when others have reached out to me for ideas. They are extremely similar to the roommate situations I've outlined above for parents of children with special needs.

If my primary caregiver, who also pays most of the bills, passed away suddenly, my living situation would be rendered more precarious as a result of their passing. This would include a large monthly mortgage; bills for water, transit, electricity, gas and so on would have to be paid; and I could not afford all of that. I would become the support person parent figure in a dorm-like setting that I outlined in the other example. In a four-bedroom house, perhaps I'd have to give up my office - and seeing as my house is already accessible for me as a wheelchair user, it would make an ideal dwelling for two, maybe three other people with disabilities as well. This was an option - but was it something I liked? I hadn't actually tried it, so I don't know. But it was important for me to just have it in mind as a potential possibility, which in turn permitted me to remain in a place with which I was already familiar - not to mention that already had all the equipment and mobility adaptations I needed - under the least amount of stress. I'd then become a landlord and thus would have some extra responsibilities: hiring handy workers to fix this and that, learning about safety protocols, camera and alarm installations, and how to vet potential tenants to share my home.

The other option is of course to streamline expenses by

downsizing, moving to a smaller place in a less pricey area - maybe even hiring a live-in caregiver.

As a person with a disability with an accessible home, a part of me desperately wants to provide up to three afford-able/accessible living spaces for other people with disabilities; yet that venture isn't without risk. If I couldn't make that happen and had to move, I'd then be the one in search of such a set up for myself. The former roommate situation is pretty stan-dard and seems less of a headache. My point about both of the above options is that they are something to think about, they are very doable options, and they could work.

Housing, whatever that looks like in your life, will be some-thing you have to define and figure out for your own unique situation. Also, realize that it won't always be exactly what you desire or look quite like what you had in mind. Sometimes having to hire a stranger as my caregiver isn't what I desire, or having them around what can seem like all the time. At times, you may just desire to be alone, wishing you didn't have to need any assistance at all. If you live alone already, sometimes you may wish you had someone around to talk to, to be there, to do small things you may need done around the house that you cannot physically do. These will be mainstays, whether you are a person with a disability or not. These are issues and feelings that come and go and some you can't get around at all.

Through all of this, choice is the main thing. The group home setting has changed and evolved. The range of home supports available through programs such as home- and community-based care has expanded, with the realization that in-home care is vital to one's wellbeing and quality of life. Accessible, affordable spaces are increasing, and advocacy for still more is needed to bring about the level of inventory and change we need as a community.

In the previous chapter, I talked about ideal living access to the things you need, and where to look to see how people with disabilities fare in various locales. The problem with this data is that it's segmented on various data points that include income, transportation, education, disease, plus things you can find almost anywhere – that is, schools, colleges and universities, and crime reports. What I think is a better indicator for evaluating potential areas to live, when coupled with the information sources above, is the presence of people with disabilities overall, and the accompanying supports in the community offering programs and services. I've mentioned that I work for one of four hundred Centers for Independent Living, also called CILs. There are a number of them, and, with so many throughout the United States, some are naturally better than others. As well as the existence of a CIL in the area, another important question is where does the majority of their funding come from? All CILs receive some type of federal funding, and that amount will likely be based on prevalence of people with disabilities per locale.

Other factors I would think about are:

- What other funders do they have? How much do they fund?
- Does the Governor's office, City Council or other official state agency offer funding in addition to federal funding? What's the fundraising strategy like and is there a robust network of givers? For me, additional funding support beyond government means there is real buy-in from those offices.
- What neighboring counties fund that particular center?

Most of this information will be a matter of public record. Another important resource is talking to actual center staff, to ask them what their own issues and drawbacks are about living where they do as a person with a disability. What do they do at the center?; what other programs do they offer, and what exciting changes are happening in the area on policy fronts such as the ADA? What kinds of specific disabilities do they serve or have a high percentage of? Additionally, I would check out websites for the area. What other nonprofit organizations are either headquartered there or have chapter offices there? What needs were those other nonprofits created to address?

While most all CILs offer the same five core services, many have additional programs that differ from state to state, or those that were created to answer a specific need in the community. For example, an equipment recycle program or loan closet program - the type I mentioned in the chapter on Recreation - might have been created because there was a prevalence of folks who did not qualify for Medicaid programs, or because there is no Medicaid, meaning that lack of jobs meant no income for Durable Medical Equipment (DME). We too have a DME recycle program - however, it's largely stocked by local people who do have quality medical insurance, good government jobs and an ability to get new equipment every few years, because of what their insurance is willing to pay for. To be frank, another source of quality medical equipment is death. While jarring, the reality is that families of people with disabilities who pass away are aware of CILs existence, so rather than put such quality and expensive equipment in the trash and fill up local landfills, they know they can put it in the hands of someone who desperately needs it.

Our own center's issue is, in fact, that the large number of people with disabilities living in the local area and the wide availability of government jobs can sometimes even cause a surplus of equipment that we cannot accept due to our own limited storage space. We are constantly turning over equipment after cleaning or addressing minor repairs, such as new batteries or tire replacement. While I wish every nonprofit could take all the donated equipment out there, please make an effort to still donate it even if a non-profit turns it down. You can always post on Facebook Marketplace or Craigslist to list items for free and get it out to the community where you live.

What other things do you need in order to make where you will choose to live an ideal place? Here are a few more of mine:

- Doctors willing to permit me to remain in my wheelchair to complete certain procedures, e.g. eye and dental exams. This isn't so much about location as it is about a can-do attitude by medical professionals. From calling around, I have seen some medical facilities that are simply unwilling to make the accommodation. However, it can be an issue of location. Limited choice implies there are only a few selections available, as in a small or rural town. It may even indicate that a popular doctor would not have to take me if he/she believes I'll require additional accommodations.
- A DME service provider and dealer, to get me fitted for new wheelchairs when I need to be. Through many medical insurance companies, you can have new equipment - including wheelchairs - every 4-7 years, as they do not last very long. Such a dealer can also repair other types of DME you may have.
- Same for my accessible vehicle. The expense and

complexity of the hand controls means a dwindling number of installers and specialists are equipped with the knowledge and tools to repair my car. Most chain or privately-owned mechanics won't even touch specialized equipment, due to liability issues. As a result, modified vehicle providers often cluster around cities and urban areas with a greater concentration of people with disabilities who need their services.

CIL is a peer run model of service, unlike any other public, government-funded program. For this reason, talking with CIL staff can be a great resource for helping you gauge what the community is like: what successes are being had in that community, how gainfully employed people with disabilities are faring in the community, and whether the area has reached various levels of progress in the key areas that are important to you. Whatever your housing set-up will be, choice should be paramount; but safety, community access and affordability are equally important factors you'll have to keep in mind as you search for the perfect set-up that's right for you.

Remember: even what seems ideal from afar might not be so stellar when you take out the microscope and start to dig deeper. An area next to a large, diverse university hospital might seem the place to be for those with chronic illness, until you find that most graduates who get training there don't actually take professional positions in that area because the earnings are too low, opting instead for the hustle and bustle of an urban area. A place closer to the city often presents a smog and pollution problem that increases the amount of irritants for those who have respiratory disabilities, so that may strike it off your list.

I have been in the position of gathering data to make a relocation decision. At the time, I was investigating a certain Southern state in which to make my new home. On calling some very helpful staff at the local CIL, I was shocked to find that their Center had a program similar to one where I lived. The cost of living is exponentially cheaper, by at least $20K; but the income this staffer could obtain and still get home care assistance by the state, was around $25,000. This might not mean anything until you learn that in the other location to which I was thinking about moving, people with disabilities could make up to $50,000 and still receive state assistance to pay for home care. That's nearly half. After the $50,000 income mark, one would need to pay some, perhaps even all of their home care expenses out of pocket. Don't forget, there are additional supplies and materials needed on top of the base price of having caregivers.

This example should illustrate how costly it can be to simply exist as a person with a disability, coupled with the trappings of a high priced area. If you require assistance to live your daily life, it will be important to review these aspects extra closely.

These are just some of the details that you'll want to find out about that impact on what you can afford, costs of living and your overall economic health.

Well before Millennial's made living at home with their parents so popular, the truth for me was that I always saw myself living in a two-bedroom condominium in the Northern Virginia area. I'm not saying that it wasn't doable to live alone, but as a person with a disability, I would always have had numerous obstacles to overcome. Safety, access to a good pool of applicants to provide personal care, and the need for multiple public transit options are all critical. Additionally, the sad reality is that there can be such a high turnover rate in the home care business, not to mention the chronic no-shows that occur and the difficulty of finding a back-up at the last minute. All of this, coupled with the high price of city living, amenities, parking, HOA fees and so forth, can mean that as you mature, you take the opportunity to find out what's truly important to you and what's most practical. These revelations can cause you to reevaluate and relax those particular standards you had previously thought were ideal.

Meager housing availability and dwindling numbers of caregiver jobs seem all the more dire when coupled with the number of aging Americans, people with disabilities and a number of other socioeconomic factors. We can guess that these factors will eventually create some pretty calamitous situations. Ensuring that your location affords you the greatest chance at success within the facets of your life that matter the most to you is key. This is about more than the costs of living: it also involves progressive attitudes from those in position of power to grant access, as well as the general thoughts of those in leadership. Ultimately, it's about knowing that government assistance programs such as social security disability cannot provide what you need to live without some sort of supplemental income from other sources. In many cases, this knowledge extends to the certainty that assistance from family and relatives or a substantial windfall like the lottery will be necessary to get by in a comfortable manner.

If you do have public assistance and benefits and currently reside with family, look into special needs trusts and other forms of financial planning for the future. You'll want to ensure that any assets left to you won't count against you and/or negatively impact your important benefits for the long term. You'll need to speak to an experienced attorney about these programs to get them securely in place.

Whatever your housing arrangement ends up being, so long as you are happy with it and it works for you, that's all that will matter.

TAKE ACTION ON HOUSING

- Before deciding where you want to live, think about WHAT you need first. This can expedite weeding out possible results that just won't work.
- As the national initiatives director of The National Arc said, thinking outside the box is key. You are only as limited as your thinking, and if you can conceptualize something, chances are you can see it through to fruition. While you're having these awesome thoughts, the only considerations you'll want to be extremely careful about are around safety. Unscrupulous characters prey on people with disabilities because our unique needs and vulnerabilities are real. With horror stories aplenty, be certain to talk with others to help test and flesh out your ideas before implementing them.
- While only in Minnesota at this time, the Rumi Program (a play on "roommate" - https:// meetmyrumi.com/), similar programs are being developed in multiple locations across the US. Rumi's model matches caregivers with people with

disabilities who receive home- and community-based programs. Although they are all called something different, similar iterations include Friendship House in Michigan, tied to a theological Seminary; Duke Divinity School in North Carolina; Vanderbilt University in Tennessee; and George Fox University in Oregon. Another Friendship House is planned for Fayetteville, N.C., to bring students studying for health care careers together with people with disabilities.

- Several colleges and universities have efforts similar to this type of partnership: George Mason University in Virginia, for example, has programs for students with intellectual and developmental disabilities that give them the college life experience, learning training and job skills while also living in dorms on campus and taking part in some regular classes with their nondisabled peers. As the need for these inclusive experiences grows, I believe more state colleges and universities, even community colleges, trade and technical schools, will eventually implement similar programmatic experiences, ensuring that people with disabilities have the opportunity to live on their own away from home, fully integrated with their peers, who are also the ones to provide care and behavior supports.

- Home is a place where you have control, can be sheltered, obtain everything you need and be safe. While those models look different for everyone, disabled or not, take some time while your current living conditions are stable to talk with friends, caregivers and relatives and make a plan: not only for the future, but for the theoretical scenario in which some or all of your carefully orchestrated foundation takes a hit, making your situation more precarious. This type of planning is just as crucial as your funeral wishes and your desires for the handling of your estate. Plans and possibilities need to be thought out, however: possible events such as sudden illness, stroke, or COVID can ultimately create stressful situations and really reduce the amount of time you have to get things in place. Your best planning time is right now.

- On a related note, even as you read this, your family may well have thoughts and ideas of their own about the best course of action for your life. They may even have given it more thought than you have. They may have you all set up to live with someone in the future who you would personally think is the last person on earth they should put you with. Full and frank communication about your personal desires, wants and needs now will minimize confusion, hurt feelings and missteps when it's time to make moves.

- I think that as people with disabilities, there are many models that are vastly different from person to person and as such might not look how you intended when introduced into your own life. What is important is that you have the access and the freedom to do the things that you want.

- Check The National Arc, Centers for Independent Living and other grassroots disability-focused organizations to find out what kind of programs exist near you.

- Some important considerations that I did not address fully in this chapter but that remain tremendously important in your housing considerations include: housing prices, climate impact, propensity and frequency of natural disasters, extreme heat or cold weather, flooding, availability of systems assisting people with disabilities in the event of a regional or national emergency that causes displacement and evacuation, personal property taxes and tax relief, median income levels, poverty levels, retirement living options, air quality, drivability (e.g. hilly vs. flat streets in neighborhoods), gas prices, crime rates - including sex offender registries and the disclosure practices of such information, getting around, conducting background checks, registries for criminal offenders, laws concerning caregiver abuse and financial abuse, a city or town being bike friendly (often meaning there is a prevalence of limited-mobility-friendly pathways and plenty of sidewalks and trails to get around town easily), the availability of bus and train, Metrorail and inner city lite-rail transit systems, schools, neighborhoods with better schools and graduation rates (higher priced home inventory, but also indicates the presence of more young people to help out and possibly build relationships with), demographic data which includes racial diversity, age and relationship status. *There's no such thing as too much information (TMI) when it comes to finding the right place to live.*

- Comparing data across all these areas will allow you to make a more informed decision about how well your individual needs will be met in each state. For example, I do drive, but when extensive repairs are needed, the service has had to keep my vehicle for an extended period of time: once, I was kept waiting seven weeks without transportation. This was devastating – plus, who knows if driving will always be accessible to me? Thus, back-up options will be something I'm always thinking about. If you can easily transfer yourself to any friend or neighbor's car, and your chair is easily folded into a backseat or trunk, then transit won't be something you are quite as concerned about. If you have regular insurance through your employer, moving to a state with no Medicare providers won't be as big a deal, but what if you can't find a job, lose it or are furloughed? For many, Medicare isn't an option. Some states have few to no Medicare providers; and an area with few medical doctors that accept Medicare could mean expensive travel to neighboring areas or even another state entirely to get medical attention.

- In some areas, under IRS guidelines, the income of caregivers providing disability services in their own home is tax-free – although there are some caveats to this and you will need to check state rules and regulations.

- The below site provides a map based on various aspects I've discussed above, outlining the best and worst states for people with disabilities. While it has some very low ranking states, you'll have to interpret that data as it pertains to your unique perspective. For instance, many Southeastern states in this survey found themselves in the lowest reaches of all 50. States in the Northeast, Midwest, and Pacific Northwest ranked higher. Whatever the ranking, remember the information is subjective and may be about data points you care little about and that have no bearing on your disability whatsoever. With all this in mind, the five states that received the highest ranking are: 1. Massachusetts 2. Pennsylvania, 3. Vermont, 4. North Dakota, and 5. Maryland. *See the full article by Derek Silva at Policygenius, dated June 2019, here: https://www.policygenius.com/disability-insurance/the-best-states-for-living-with-a-disability/*

- There are a number of sources for home or environmental modifications in order to increase accessibility options in your home. These programs range from one-time grants that do not need to be paid back to low-to-no-interest loans. Check with state and local county government to find out more about these programs. Note that some programs will only be available depending on the year the property was built and that different programs will apply to renters and owners. Keep in mind that some changes made to a rental property may need to be returned to their original conditions before moving.

- Tax credits and incentives also exist for making

modifications within residences and/or public facilities. For example, if you need to ask your landlord about installing a ramp, hand rails, grabber bars or other environmental modifications, reading up on state incentives for such changes can encourage to them to get it done. Also consult tax professionals, your own preparer and the IRS for more information.

- Knowing Your Housing Rights is a complex but important document that you should read and try to understand as much as possible prior to starting parts of your housing search. The Department of Justice (DOJ) and the Department of Housing and Urban Development (HUD) are jointly responsible for enforcing the federal Fair Housing Act. View more information about what they do, here: https://www.justice.gov/crt/us-department-housing-and-urban-development

- Living on your own may not look as you intended and that's okay. You have to define a personal level of success. Always remember that safety is paramount. Caregivers don't always take your needs seriously and may leave you without backup, sometimes calling to say they cannot come at the very last minute. This is the harsh reality to deal with and to plan around. It's also why having a network, building relationships and establishing back-up plans for your back-up plan are crucial to your success.

- Look into various security measures if you do require assistance. You could talk to a safety expert and a SMART Home Specialist (also called Home

Automation Consultants) who can help you figure out systems and products that are best to meet your needs. These will not only give you peace of mind but automate tasks, making it easier for you live where you choose.

7 / RECREATION

Key Takeaways

- Recreation of all the vast types of programs for people with disabilities has tremendously evolved, giving us more access and inclusion to everything others could never have dreamed of us participating in even just twenty years ago.
- Access to programs is paramount. If it doesn't exist where you live, find a model program and replicate it locally. People are more than willing to help you get your version off the ground. You simply need to find even a handful of folks who are also desiring this program, to help you get it off the ground.
- Recreation outlets are a vital part of good physical and mental health and are not SOLELY about exercise and agility.
- Think outside the box for your own "recreational pursuits" e.g. crafting, handiwork, civic, religious, ministry participation, and things done indoors,

outdoors or wherever. Community engagement and opportunities to demonstrate your ability to plan and lead -if it makes you feel a part of something is engaging and challenging and fun, there's no reason it can't fit in your definition of recreation.

- With the previous bullet, do not let service-type opportunities fall under the guise of recreation. In an advocacy role, as people with disabilities, our desire to contribute to the world around us and to demonstrate our abilities and knowledge can mask as recreation when in truth, it's arduous work. The once fun outlet of organizing can become burdensome. Others may look to you to fulfill a role, and then you may feel the need to step up, falsely believing this is your only valuable contribution to society. Your worth can get wrapped up in doing things rather than the personal joy you once found from said activities.

To say that recreation for people with disabilities has evolved since I was a child is the understatement of the year. Still, in an elementary school that had a wonderful and robust physical education component, even as a person with a disability, PE was fun.

I can remember being placed on a carpeted board with wheels, almost like a skateboard but wider, and using my arms to pull myself around the entire gym. All of us with mobility issues were on these boards and moving around, many of us quite fast, narrowly missing each other. Like I said, it was fun!

These boards were the brainchild of one of the first few PE teachers I would be fortunate enough to encounter who really made the effort to adapt our recreation, before that was a thing.

Rather than look at children with disabilities and say "*I don't know what to do here*," these great teachers were willing and creative enough to suggest trying this or that. I even remember being placed on a trampoline, just sitting there, unable to move or jump around a lot myself, as the teacher bounced in the center, lifting all of us gathered around. This was thrilling to me: all of us wheelchair users out of our chairs and on this black mesh netting, with the zany teacher jumping as hard as she could to lift us all into the air with the residual bounce. *How did she even think this would work?* is my first thought now as an adult - that and *how did she know we'd find such exhilarating joy in the process*? How did she know how important any movement and participation at all would be to us?

This was adaptive recreation in the purest form: a heart-led thing, all about seeing what could be done, rather than all the science that might take issue with the details of exactly how teachers went about their inclusive practices, limiting their rather 'duct-tape' approach. I could see how science and doctors of yesteryear might have limited many teacher's first ideas, leaving children with disabilities out of the mix entirely, and thus leading them to miss out on this fun experience.

That's part of the issue I see today. There are two sides, really: those that get the children fully involved and others with the mindset, "no, that's too dangerous, so let's not do anything in the recreation department whatsoever."

The thing about recreation isn't at all about the whys and wherefores of what's being done. It's about the inclusiveness of it all: the opportunity to rest from your normal academics or work pursuits simply for the enjoyment that something brings. Merriam Webster defines Recreation as *refreshment of strength and spirits after work; also, a means of refreshment or diversion.* Other definitions include "activity done for enjoyment when one is not working" and "athletic and recreation facilities".

What's important to understand about recreation is that it doesn't always mean physical activity but simply something you engage in and enjoy doing.

I'm so thankful for having had the opportunity to join some of the things I can remember getting involved in as a child. One of these was Muscular Dystrophy (MD) camp, where we not only had physical activities included as part of our day, but other things: campfires, arts and crafts, talent night. These are also recreation, so we should definitely remove the notion that only physical activity is recreation. Just because you're not doing any major physical activity - and you won't often break a sweat when you whip out your glue gun – you'll still be having fun, engaging with others and gaining the opportunity to share and show your strengths and abilities, as well as enjoying opportunities for fun, relationships, fellowship and camaraderie.

Another means of recreation for people with disabilities that is admittedly also part work is on the advocacy fronts with which many of us find ourselves involved. Many people with disabilities have found their voice and felt a part of something within state, regional and national level politics and policymaking. In the earlier chapter on Advocacy, I talked about the program with the sole goal of raising up the next generation of leaders to create change for people with disabilities and their families - exactly what the Partners in Policymaking program was all about. However, take it from someone who has been doing those things since my teens (that's almost thirty years): don't let those your advocacy volunteering become overly burdensome. Yes, I get it, you'll find you enjoying those opportunities to participate, contribute to your world and make a real difference, tremendously; but be cautious not to throw yourself into this role 24/7 and eventually face burnout.

Early in my own advocacy journey, service was a way to be included, and, if I'm brutally honest, also to posture: a platform from which to articulate, showing and sharing the knowledge I possessed, as well as a surefire way to add to my resume, fit in and gain acceptance and respect from my peers in the meantime.

Somewhere along the way, however, no matter how much I enjoyed it, it was almost like I couldn't exist without it. At that point, it became real work. Nervous of ever finding myself isolated, I was always serving in my community: secretary, chair, vice chair, event planning committee chair and ministry lead at church, and on and on. This causes burnout and then it's not any kind of *"refreshment of strength and spirits **after work**"*... it *is* work! I began to feel labeled by what I was doing and what role I fulfilled, rather than just being appreciated and having the fun of participation. I personally think this is a pitfall that all people, regardless of ability levels, can fall into; yet I do feel it occurs for more people with disabilities because there are so few recreational choices, especially as one ages. Couple that with sometimes dwindling mobility, lack of transit and access and the only remaining option, it can seem, is that of advocacy work.

What I will say is that for people with disabilities, myself included, it's hard to find something as you age. Getting into something that gives you a true feeling of having fun, of being exhausted by working hard yet also liberated: that addictive feeling other folks get when they do a sport, or engage in any competitive contact event, where it's a battle of wills, skills or strength.

For me, service – taken on to fit in and give myself something to do - was supposed to be some kind of "after-work activity". Yet, however hard I tried to put it under the "recreation" category, it was really not. Take heed that anything can turn into work, even if you love it. Volunteerism is a worthwhile thing, but it too can become burdensome: free labor that you can began to resent.

When talking about recreation, ask yourself: are you feeling included? Are you building real friendships not built on some kind of expectation to perform; and, most importantly, are you having FUN? Are you feeling expended energy (not exhausted) in a good way?

Looking back on service positions and the volunteerism with which I've been involved over the years, some of those relationships didn't translate into folks I hung out with outside of the volunteer time - and that's the problem. These opportunities should build friendships and long-lasting relationships outside of just coming together for a common goal. Many women, especially, talk about how difficult it is to build and maintain relationships later in life. That's because we're all busy doing something: working, family, working, and more working, even in a volunteer position.

Today, there is almost no sport in existence that hasn't been somehow modified for people with disabilities by someone. If you felt that lots of things done by your nondisabled peers throughout school were out of your reach, this is probably another reason it's so hard to find what it is you like to do now: many of the modifications have only come about in the last ten years. If you doubt that, ask the Paralympian archery champion Matt Stutzman. He uses his feet as he was born without arms, to both raise and pull back the bow of his bow and arrow and while he can walk, he's seated to do this.

We can all learn to adapt whatever we want to do, to create a custom-made recreational outlet just for us. Now, I'm fairly sure I won't qualify for the Paralympics, but watching and understanding the ways in which athletes with similar disabilities have made adaptations to almost any sport should be encouraging to us all. We will all be better for trying and finding different ways and means.

The Paralympics has at least 40 types of sport/competitive categories, including:

Archery
    Athletics (include wheelchair racing and club throw)
    Badminton
    Boccia (ball sport, involves throwing the ball farthest distance)
    Canoeing
    Cycling (track and road)
    Equestrian
    Football
    Judo
    Powerlifting
    Rowing
    Shooting
    Swimming
    Table tennis
    Triathlon (added in 2020)
    Volleyball

Wheelchair basketball

Wheelchair fencing

Wheelchair rugby

Wheelchair tennis

This list is simply a place to draw from, but it's far from all-inclusive of everything recreation can encompasses. "Sport" alone can mean water sports, arts and crafts, campfires, horseback riding - and, believe it or not, there are even rock climbers with disabilities ascending some of our greatest natural mountains right from their wheelchairs.

Recreation is anything that you want it to be. Hopefully you had the privilege of being taught at school by some of the talented adaptive recreation folks we have today. I sincerely hope that helped you continue on a path that will serve you into adulthood and old age.

Sadly, though, adaptive recreation is an increasingly rare thing in K-12 systems. Of course, it then becomes something for which you have to pay, sometimes steeply, as you age. By that time, those muscles have atrophied and the stigma is real, expressed through staring and curiosity from strangers. This sort of curiosity, despite showing the admirable desire to know more in a healthy way, can nonetheless make you feel like an oddity simply for trying to do something that's important to your health.

I realize some of this sounds so depressingly dismal. My point is that those teachers, the Kennedy Family that created the Special Olympics, those that built the modified bowling assistance ramp and eventually created the Paralympics: all of these people's work sends the important message that we can and should strive to keep doing something, regardless of limitation. Even people with disabilities were not meant for inactivity, regardless of the severity.

Now, some history. A German doctor named Ludwig Guttmann, a pre-World War II neurologist and champion of the belief that sport could be a method of rehabilitation for people with disabilities, started "Parasport". In July 1948, Guttman established the Stoke Mandeville Games to coincide with the 1948 Olympic games in London and brought about the first parasport competitive event for wheelchair athletes.

If you really think about the atmosphere immediately following the world wars, the men likely needed something to get them going. Feeling dejected and "less-than" after injury – a feeling relatable to many of us due to our limits, both self-inflicted and imposed by an oppressive society - the men who acquired disabilities during the war may have felt like mere shells of what they considered normal, healthy and even virile. Thus, the addition of sport provided a way for them to reengage, bringing about some normalcy and healthy competition. The fact that they played against others with similar disabilities meant the playing field was proportionate, making it a true competition, not only of strength but also seeing the various ways in which different people adapted to their disabilities. How fortunate we are to have so many willing models, doctors and builders who all sought to improve things, believing that with some modification, participation could be made a reality for many who were previously cast aside and effectively left for dead. People with disabilities have always had that ability to adapt. Finding healthy ways to make recreation accessible should be no different.

To find healthy physical outlets, similarly to good mental health outlets as addressed in my other chapter, these type of people are your go to. Therapists, occupational and physical, as well as doctors are good places to talk through possible exercise regimens that would work for you, as well as trainers who have experience with people with disabilities; and of course, other peers with disabilities.

Online, there is a directory of personal trainers who self-report their experience and qualifications for working with clients with disabilities and health conditions. This is part of the National Center on Health, Physical Activity and Disability (NCHPAD), working to connect people with disabilities to fitness instructors and professional trainers in your community who either have existing experience or may be looking to expand their client base to people with a variety of need levels and abilities. See a link to their information in the Index.

It is this can-do attitude that you will need to look for in life to assist you and/or your young child with a disability. We also had a heated pool in my elementary school of almost 40 years ago, although sadly I haven't seen one since. When I think about those awesome times, I can't help but compare them to my junior high and high school experiences. There, by contrast, there wasn't much of anything: you could basically opt out of anything that challenged you physically. Well, within that type of framework, there goes your entire mindset about fitness! Besides that, there were of course the physical and bodily changes and the universal devil of comparison to others that keeps so many people from venturing to other places to start an exercise regimen. Then the pounds pack on as a result: the perfect accessory to go with that awkward teenage acne, not to mention everything else. Those adolescent years can so easily shape that sedentary lifestyle, and you might not much care again until you're almost middle aged. Well, it's not that you don't care – of course you do – but it's hard to know what to do when you lack access to a more regimented adaptive exercise program, especially when the creative folks you once knew who cared about your participation are no more. YOU have to care!

This determination to do something, to participate and get involved, is going to be on you, no excuses. There now exist a number of opportunities to take part, get motivated and get out there again. I can't say that folks won't stare and nearly fall off their own exercise equipment checking you out to see how you do it (this is the voice of personal experience speaking). You do have to work to get past that if you want to participate in public options. If you don't, there are still online exercise groups that you can do at home in private, some even free. Additionally, there are lots of groups out there. Even physical therapy is a way to get prepared, for which your doctor can often write you a prescription. Insurance may pay for some if not all of it. On a related note, you can set up a consultation, often free, with a nutritionist: a doctor can refer you, or you can often find these resources at some of the larger grocery stores and in-store pharmacies.

At minimum, you can always do basic range-of-motion exercises to keep yourself flexible and limber. Reach out to speak with your doctor about such questions. Often, an experienced caregiver will also know how to do these: they're usually included as part of their training and if you let them know, they can assist you too. You never know what knowledge caregivers possess. I've found many who often started in cosmetology or hospitality jobs that enhance their skillsets and thus their ideas to your benefit. I know this because mine asks me about exercise all the time, even though I pay her not to!

Recreation isn't just about physical recreation but also mental agility, holistic well-being and inclusive communities, which I'll talk about later in this chapter and touch on again in the chapter on housing. As I mentioned, the National Center on Health, Physical Activity and Disability (NCHPAD) is a resource that identifies a number of recreational resources for people with disabilities. To see what is available both nationally and internationally, visit www.nchpad.org. These resources include such things as organization directories, adaptive fitness and recreation programs, accessible facilities, assistive technology and equipment vendors, plus a number of links to journal articles, books, videos and more. Fact sheets are available on a variety of activities, targeted toward people with disabilities, fitness professionals, health professionals and researchers.

There is no age minimum or maximum to change your outlook on your health, your access to others for support, information and advice, or to improve your physical and mental fitness. In the Take Action Section, as well as in the index, resources and Quick Guide, we also list a few free internet-based fitness and nutrition programs in which you can take part.

Of course, even with the advancements to all forms of life and access to living through the signing of the ADA, the reality is that inaccessibility still exists, from leisure to recreation facilities to aviation and international travel. This lack of access still makes it difficult to get around, and some areas are still not completely accessible. Companies that are not fully ADA-compliant can make it difficult to work, have fun and enjoy your life.

There are a number of studies that evaluate the quality of life and living experienced by people with disabilities around the world, based on certain data. Even if you're able to relocate geographically, though, let's face it: moving is so often not an option. Even if you do, there's no guarantee that the same issues you face around accessibility won't be similar in another locale.

There just aren't any guarantees on anything, especially when it comes to people with disabilities. Another issue with the data gathered through such surveys is that who even knows the type of people they interviewed for it? They could very well have found people with disabilities to ask, but these people may or may not be gainfully employed, may or may not be able to afford the costs of living where they are, due to the amount of available gainful and competitive job opportunities, not to mention good jobs and supports in the academic setting. A balmy year-round climate in the south may be a wonderful thing to have and soothing on one's muscles, but if there is a high level of poverty and few jobs in such areas, what use is the great weather if you're sitting at home with paltry funds in your pocket? At least you don't then have to also spend money on winter attire, right? You get the idea.

Here are some places to look and some aspects of life to think about as you try your best to orchestrate a life that has all the elements you desire, making it a live worth living with access to the things you really need.

Centers for Disease Control

- Look for data on health disparities.

- Insurance costs, and Medicaid/Medicare availability.

- Public health systems and grades for care.

- Large universities and/or medical facilities in the area near where you will live.

Census Bureau data

- Income/annual earnings for people with/without disabilities.

- Average household incomes.

Education

- School grades/averages.

- Number of schools, and graduates.

- Number of teachers in the area and average teacher income. Do teachers live in the area themselves or do they commute due to lack of adequate/affordable housing?

- Number of recreation centers, summer jobs for youth, and other availability of youth activity centers and sports programs.

Policing / Crime Data

- Number and types of incidents.

- Drug usage data, which also correlates to the availability of jobs.

Policygenius -

- Finally, Policygenius has created an index that paints a picture of which states are more livable for Americans with disabilities. Using the most recent data available, including the latest government-reported data, they compare all 50 states and Washington, D.C., across more than two dozen factors on their website. Their factors include:

- **economic data** , including income and the unemployment rate for residents with a disability

- **affordability** , including housing costs as a percent of income

- **livability** , how easy it is for residents to get around

- the state of **health care** and insurance

I'll talk more about these in the next chapter on Housing, which may seem a more appropriate chapter to delve into such topics, but hopefully by beginning to think about all of these aspects you can correlate how the availability of some opportunities and access to quality of living, can enhance or significantly restrict your quality of living and yes, your access to recreation and leisure.

TAKE ACTION ON RECREATION

- When your doctor asks you those standard wellness questions and even on normal visits, share your concerns about being able to locate physical and mental health / fitness supports. They may have ideas that can assist you. What's more, they may have patients with similar issues that have been able to find help for themselves.

- While I think it's important to share your issues with your doctor, I also realize that some still adhere to a model of medicine that makes them rather limited and ignorant about their prognosis for people with disabilities. If this is your experience, find new medical practitioners. You deserve to see practitioners who are more aware, open to new ways of thinking and willing to both hear about, try, recommend and even prescribe what you need. Note: As mentioned above, it's possible to have PT prescribed as a medical need and thus have insurance pay for it. Even some equipment can be prescribed by doctors to benefit your life and well-being, opening up ways to pay for these lifesaving tools. When I use the word "prescribe" here, I'm not necessarily referring to medication, although that can certainly be a vital tool in your overall health goals too.

- We need to reduce our tendency to categorize our disabilities into too many separate boxes. When compared one to another, we often find that many disabilities have similar ailments, and manifest themselves in parallel ways, though they have completely different diagnoses. As a result, we can find more treatments that work and similar remedies, through experience sharing. If your specific disability organization doesn't have resources related to certain issues that you are facing, don't be afraid to look around at others. While not all will be helpful, perhaps because you don't have the specific diagnosis to meet their criteria for service, some of things they recommend and many of the support groups to which they can at minimum refer you won't be as restrictive. By talking with them, you may find the information you need.

- Many organizations have loan closets. This is a wonderful resource to inquire about. In the loan closet, there is equipment available that someone donated, usually after death, or because they only needed it temporarily. Rather than discard a very expensive piece of equipment, the loan closet stores it and can loan it out to interested parties. One way this could work, for example, is that if you wanted to go swimming at your local pool, the facility may not have an extra pool chair (one that can get wet without rusting) for you to use. You obviously cannot use your own chair as it may become damaged, but the loan closet may have something they can give you to keep at the facility, locked in their storage - so you don't have to transport it back and forth - and get it out for you each time you need to use it, in order to take advantage of aquatic exercise.

- Find the right lingo and be specific! There is nothing wrong with discussing the core of what ails you. Being honest and candid with the right people will get you the best answers and results. Sometimes when we are too embarrassed to address something directly, this causes confusion and can lead you to the wrong thing, causing frustration and wasted time. Find out the proper terminology so you can better describe and discuss issues with those who are in a position to help you.

- Even a disease or type of disability that has a very small group of affected people , e.g. only 100 folks in the United States have what you have, that is still 99 people that have likely felt the desire to come together to discuss it. Sometimes, if you don't find folks that share the issues you experience, do not be afraid to start the very kind of group that you need yourself.

- Do not let age deter you from locating a program or group of supportive people to help you address your physical and mental health issues. There can be a bit of a program participation desert for those of us with disabilities who are aged 28-55. While this is unfortunate, we are a growing demographic and as such, there are a number of burgeoning resources being realized to address the lack of programs for us. Watch this space.

- The program "A Healthier You" provides information on nutrition and exercise, with motivational tools for choosing new, healthy behaviors available at the NCHPAD.

- Just as uncovering information can sometimes feel like finding a golden needle in a haystack, remember that others like you are also seeking this information, resources and knowledge. Try to share what you've learned with others. You don't have to write a book (hehe) but Facebook groups, online clearinghouses, forums and message boards, plus social media platforms (maybe even your own YouTube Channel, you never know!) are wonderful ways to share information through a post that can eventually be seen by millions of people.

8 / CAREGIVING

KEY TAKEAWAYS

- Finding quality care is possible! The world is full of kind, compassionate caregivers who have a heart for assisting people in general, and you or your loved ones in particular, in times of need.
- Try not to be too adamant about being the boss, or that this relationship can't at some point grow into a respectful friendship beyond employee/employer. Balance can be difficult but is attainable.
- Just as in any profession, there are some bad actors, but don't let one bad experience deter you from striving to find a truly lasting and respectful relationship. Great people are out there.
- Teaching children and young adults that there are more people than those related to them (Mommy, Daddy, Auntie, Grandma, etc.) that can also provide care for them is key to alleviating your superhuman complex, along with any feelings of

unhealthy guilt about your child's chronic disease. This can be a major step in your child's ability to become independent, increase self-reliance and foster their ability to ask others for help. They will also learn to rely on other people besides you, who can help them just as much as you do.

- Caregiving is a rewarding but often thankless career. There are many people who want to be the "boss" of caregivers and the tasks with which they are charged. Bear in mind that the line between caring for the main person and "work" for the rest of the family's needs should not be blurred. Added stress can all too easily be put on the caregiver, particularly when there are multiple people and/or generations in the home. High staff turnover, communication breakdowns and other issues will negatively affect the person receiving care.

- Your parents can't take care of you at the level of care you desire forever.

- Asking for help - as any person, disabled or not, must do at some point in their lives - shouldn't be stigmatized.

- Teach kids early and often about the qualities of good people. We should all be taught what to look out for, as well as how to be good managers of people: working WITH someone toward a mutually beneficially relationship, not wrestling within one built on subservience, condescension or abuse.

- It is easier to relax rules and to be less stringent gradually, as you and a caregiver's relationship grows. Conversely, it is impossible to lay down the rules after you've already tolerated every kind of behavior under the sun.

- Repeat: you cannot get tough and lay down the law after things have fallen apart. Be direct, command the treatment you deserve right from the interview, through the hiring process, into the maintenance of this new relationship. Too lax from the beginning and trying to change your demeanor part way through can send mixed messages and cause confusion, negative experiences and hurt feelings. It can also turn the relationship into one where you are no longer the boss.

To say that I have a long history with receiving care is an understatement. Looking back over my own history of personal caregivers and this wonderful, liberating, skilled yet deeply undervalued profession, I know I've been fortunate with what I received. However, that doesn't mean I haven't met some real characters and even had some bad experiences. What I would stress most is just dealing with the day and starting this journey. First, you have to come to terms with your limitations. I don't know anyone who feels like: "Yay, hiring a caregiver, how exciting!"

Originally, I had not even planned to include caregiving in this book. I have an entire book on caregiving that I hope to share with you in the future, but I did want to touch on some of that here too – so get ready for some spoilers! Like other chapters in this book, this will give you just a snapshot, talking about why it's so important to have care and dealing with some of the recurring issues that keep people from finding the support they need. (Alternatively, some even stop seeking professional care entirely after a few negative incidents, only to unfairly place their daily needs on family, most often aging parents.) I know it's difficult; I understand. However, it's also important to realize your family simply cannot assist you forever. As bitter a pill that is to swallow, it's a realization that you have to come to terms with. Seeing parents age right before your eyes is hard - and what's more, there's really nothing you can do to stop it.

I remember one Sunday morning my mother telling me something that was difficult to understand at first, but that would eventually be a great lesson. It wasn't what I wanted to hear at that moment, but it was more important than I can express for a child's ultimate development. Dare I say that this conversation with Mom influenced the level of independence I carried with me into adulthood. It was a blessing that this lesson was given to me at all.

To set the scene, there were a bunch of people at our house. They were visiting: I don't remember for what exactly, maybe someone's Christening or an Easter service, I've really no recollection of the occasion. The house was quite busy with activity. Everyone was rushing around getting ready, getting dressed. I was already dressed: because I took a little longer, my parents often took time to get me together and mostly set for the day, especially when folks were visiting. Both my parents grew up with a number of siblings: my dad had twelve (yes, 12! Not a typo!) and my Mom, there were seven of them. When you're young and one of two children, you never really grasp the order and precision of a well-running family and how efficiently things go, all things considered. You actually think: *OMG, what a bunch of people!* Having so many people in one house seemed like a zoo. I wasn't used to it, so it was great to find a quiet corner to wait in while everyone else got ready. The only thing left for me was to put on my shoes.

I waited patiently for my mother to help me. It's fair to say she was probably a little bit flustered, having had to cook for, clean up after and cater to the entire extended family in her house for this special event (whatever it was). It never occurred to me to ask another person to help me with my shoes. I was used to *her* assisting me, and it seemed to my young perception that I'd just wait for her. When you're used to having your mother help you, it's just a thing that naturally happens. It doesn't seem like a big deal. Finally, my poor mom got a little snippy with me and said something to the effect of: "Other people than just me can help you." It was probably more like "Do you not see all these capable people around here?" Sure I saw them, but of course I'd never considered that they were capable, or helpful, or would be willing to help me. I just didn't think at all. My approximately ten year old self really just assumed my Mother would assist me. Forever.

She was right. In hindsight, I'm appreciative of the rebuttal – although I could only make that concession as an adult – all the more so as I observe others, from little children to, yes, even some grown-ass adults, who are unwilling to accept help from someone other than their Mom and Dad.

What's sadder still is how many aging parents still cater to their adult children with disabilities, fearing... what? I don't know exactly. Some thoughts about this:

No one would ever help them the way I can!

Yes, that is true: it won't be the same. And that might be a good thing. It might just be an opportunity for your child to find his or her voice and learn to speak up.

Someone will take advantage of them...

Yes, that might be true; but it's your job to teach them the right tools to express their concern and communicate their feelings about anything unusual, not to mention the safeguards available to mitigate this risk while protecting and keeping tabs on your loved ones.

Well, I will live forever, so they will never be cared for by someone else.

Nope, that's a nice but unrealistic goal. I don't have a response to such delusion, except to remark that so many parents do secretly have this thought, only to become ill and eventually drop dead one day, leaving their child even more vulnerable because there were absolutely no plans for care put in place. Thus, nobody ever taught these individuals that there were other people who could care for and help them: that some would actually want to be of service.

Of course it was hard to ask for help. But if I ultimately wanted to learn to be independent, asking for help was par for the course. A lesson in practicing that early on would help me long-term. I found that it would become easier and easier the more I did it. I had to ask for help at the grocery store: "Excuse me, can you reach that on the shelf for me? Thanks!" Ask for help just to get *into* any store: "Can you open the door for me, please? Thanks." These may seem like trivial examples of what I'm trying to get across, but the point is that even small children learn to advocate and speak up for themselves and are already taking cues from you in some form through whatever you do. The sooner they learn this, the sooner they can become self-reliant and not have to depend on you for so much.

The important thing is to start small. An older cousin, an adult peer, a young babysitter, eventually a trained caregiver: all of these small experiences prepare them for getting along with others, speaking up and asking for assistance and thriving in an environment that won't always include Mom's or Dad's presence. They'll soon learn that it's okay to ask this person for the things they need, to help them with this or that. It's smart to begin with an hour here and there before building up to longer stretches. The longer they are together, the more trust grows as they can see someone else besides Mom and Dad in a helpful and supportive role, and the more they realize they're still alive and able to do without them.

I didn't have caregivers until I was in my twenties, and twenty plus years later, I realize that I likely didn't have to start at all. Up until then, my Mother worked a full-time job while taking care of me in the mornings and evenings every single day. I wish I could remember that first time, but I know that it was liberating. Granted, there is a learning curve! Believe it or not, though, I seemed to have a knack for reading people and I interviewed them myself, often on my own. I would interview folks back to back over the course of a few hours.

Secret tip: my Mom and I sometimes had a kind of interviewing game. She would sit in a booth next to my table and pretend to be reading the paper, from whence she could hear the entire interview. When the potential caregiver left, we'd converse about their responses to questions and she'd get to see the person. I never interview folks at my house. Even when I had to find someone during the pandemic, Zoom was a wonderful tool allowing me to maintain my anonymity and keep the less than desirable/red-flag applicants away from my door. At twenty something, it was good for me, and it helped free up my parents to do what they wanted, even to travel, with peace of mind that I would be okay in their absence.

I realize that it may all seem a bit melodramatic, as nowadays I am writing my books, speaking, working and maintaining a nine to five. All of that, however, has nothing to do with my physical abilities. My parents aren't worried about my abilities at all, but rather about medical emergencies: freak fires, burglaries, intruders outside the door and yes, for this particular example, worried about the days of intermittent no-show caregivers who don't come to work for whatever reason. While we're talking about caregivers and what a wonderful an addition they can be to any family, we have to also talk about drawbacks. A key conundrum: what to do the one time that happens if your primary care/support is halfway across the world?

So, what can you do? Answer: Back up plans for your back up plan. Some of my best caregivers have had chronically late issues, have called in sick or been ambivalent about coming to work, leaving me with little to no notice to arrange some alternative solution. And yes, that's even happened to me at the worst possible times, like when primary supports have gone out of town. It will likely happen in the course of your life, but you'll survive to realize that the benefits of support far outweigh the drawbacks.

Depending on when you start, whether as a child, youth or young adult, you can uncover so much about human beings and human potential in your child, and your child can realize resilient things in him or herself. Moreover, for younger kids, those first few short half-hours alone with caregivers can help them uncover more about the types of help to look for: the kinds of people that can fill these roles, and even why some folks might not be a good fit if you ever have to let someone go. Spoiler alert: you will have to do that. They, too, will recognize signs and likely tell you sooner, without prompting, that this isn't a good fit. Of course, you have to remember as the parent to take everything with a grain of salt, ensuring that their reasons for wanting you to terminate this person aren't simply because they can't have their way or get away with murder.

There are two instances I can recall where a caregiver

would mean so much and can really help families bettering the quality of life for the person with a disability.

The first is a man whom I'll call George. George has a young daughter with intellectual disabilities. George's daughter is almost forty years of age and George, nearing 80, has seen his own health decline due to his age. Throughout 40+ years, George has only sent the daughter to live with her Aunt, and there only for short periods of time. It's worth noting here that the Aunt can take only about two weeks of this, maximum, owing to the fact that her niece becomes belligerent over small infractions where she doesn't get her way - brought about by years of George denying her nothing.

The truth is that through the years, one caregiver after another has been "run off" by George's daughter. As time went by and the situation repeated itself, George didn't seek assistance or dig further into the problem. He simply continued letting his daughter dictate to him and get her way over and over again, till now here they are: George is aging, and what will happen to his daughter when the inevitable comes to pass? I won't elaborate on possible scenarios except to say that some may be rather unfortunate: an institution or a nursing facility, most probably, where she will have little choice over anything. Her quality of life may decline in such a place. Maybe she'll be given the opportunity to try to make it in a group home setting with peers similar in disability and age to her own; maybe her Aunt will tough it out and make it work, giving her a future of choice and family support around her until her dying days. No, we don't know what he future holds for our children with disabilities, but it's evident that there are at least some things we can take control of to ensure better security in their life path, outlining supports and preparing them to play nice with others, preventing displacement and abandonment. There are no guarantees.

I realize it's easy to give folks a pass: that what I'm saying may sound like harsh views on parents of people with ID and DD; but many people with ID and DD understand more than we think they do: about getting their way and shunning discipline. With this in mind, the perfect way doesn't exist. Small concessions will have to be made, yes, fine, but not to their detriment and safety. A life with little discipline, placating and pandering to a special needs child, won't work long term either.

Finally, another example: When I counseled a young man about living more independently, he remarked to me that when it came to care, "his mother would be taking care of him forever". He was a young male, and his paraplegia - the result of a gunshot wound to his lower torso - reminded me of the selfish nature we all can have when it comes to care. Maybe we all have that attitude toward asking for help when we don't have that experience I had at ten years of age: waiting, likely not so patiently, for my Mother to help me with my shoes.

What this says is that when we don't consciously practice self-awareness and thoughtfulness, we can fall into the same pattern. Clearly, at ten years of age, I used to have this view too: that my Mom would try to care for me forever. Doubtful. I would hope by 30 or 40 at the latest that I might have come to realize that this view is not only unrealistic but also unhealthy for both my Mom and I, as well as nearly impossible. If you don't want a caregiver for your own needs, do it because you care about those that must help you all the time without such a person around. What about dignity and privacy? I hate to say we're a selfish bunch, but here goes: from birth, we are selfish. Only at birth can we claim ignorance, and it could even be a little cute to be helpless at times growing up. Not so much when you're a full adult.

I didn't like having care at first, but I grew into it. I also realized that I could be in charge: I could come and go somewhat independently, despite living at home, if I had a caregiver that didn't mind helping me at a later hour occasionally. Likewise, if I had to get up early for something, I arranged that with my caregiver; if I wanted something moved in my room or to change anything in my own spaces, I could ask and they were there to help me. In this way, it can be liberating to have the help you need, direct your own care and be responsible for the things you need.

To return to the previous example, what I don't want is for George's daughter to be in a nursing facility: a forty-year-old hanging around seventy- and eighty-year-olds. Honestly, there are plenty of nursing facilities with young people stuck there, not because of their disability alone, but because they don't have the supports in the home within the community of their choosing. Such younger people may not know how to go about getting these supports, nor how to go about finding, hiring and managing caregivers for success: a process that many are afraid to start or don't have the technology to tackle. Another barrier, as I mentioned in the chapter on housing, is that there isn't any affordable/accessible housing in many areas – perhaps there's less inventory where you live – or maybe a smaller number of caregivers in your location who can have their pick of jobs to apply for.

In the case of the young man who is paralyzed from the waist down, he's six feet tall and probably two hundred pounds. Is it fair to his mother that she continue to be his main source of physical help? At some point, he will have to seek out additional supports in order to live the life he wants. If parents were completely honest in their roles as caregivers, most would have to admit that they have at some point lamented the hardships of care to an outsider; but have they ever addressed this issue directly with their young adult son or daughter? Such a conversation would involve alerting the adult child to the reality that their parents too could use some support? Support to care for them; support for the mental health stress aspects of the enormous amount of unpaid work; caregiver guilt and caregiver resentment... These are all real feelings that have been researched and examined that being a caregiver brings. Unfortunately, this is a taboo subject at the heart of this whole subject, and deserves a great deal of further discussion and illumination. Caregivers get burnt out, too. Aging caregivers often provide care well beyond their physical ability to do so, and can even put both themselves and their child in danger when they refuse to ask for and seek out additional help.

These situations are real. They don't work long term, and they are disasters waiting to happen. Caregivers cannot solve all problems, I understand that; but denying a need for them in your own family can set everyone up for colossal failure.

Note: I've talked extensively about care and support and the benefits they bring, but haven't said as much about the means to fund these services. Home and Community Based Services (HCBS) often pay some portion if not all of the caregiver salaries, plus some related expenses, through Centers for Medicaid and Medicare programs. Yes, some people are not able to get these services due to long waiting lists and not enough slots being offered per state, thus I realize that the services may be out of reach for some. I can only stress that you not give up.

Remember that services may be named something a little different in various locations and may fall into other pots of funding, such as the Department for Aging and Rehabilitative Services, as well as agencies specially appointed to advocate for the needs of people with disabilities. There are also new and downright revolutionary volunteer-type organizations in some situations when there are no funds for programs. The issue, however, isn't always program unavailability, but that many eligible people just don't know about these programs. Many others can be unaware of the full range of what's available: some people who may not be fully informed can include discharge planners, physical and occupational therapists, immediate care, nursing and rehabilitation centers, and others meant to assess the home situation prior to discharge – even some case managers are also unaware about what's available in the community, thus cannot share resources they don't know about. These programs, therefore, will have to be sought out through your own due diligence: by reaching out to your communities, to online groups and forums and through direct contact with your local government agencies.

Finding the right person to ask and the range of supports available is a process. As far as caregivers themselves, your very own modern-day equivalent of Florence Nightingale very may well exist - but you're going to have to shake the bushes, compromise, and teach your child to live peaceably among different types while securing their futures in order to find her.

CAREGIVING IN TIMES OF COVID

I stopped production on this book for a few reasons, but one important reason was to permit myself to expound on the unanticipated and devastatingly dramatic downturn in the availability of caregivers in COVID times.

Talk about feast to famine. A couple of things for me stood out but I wanted to add a few things most people have never thought about and don't realize, that for one, caregiving individuala's not part of an agency are considered "independent contractors." That would be great if the usual implications of "independent" and "contractor" were true. Most people think contractors are paid royally with additional funds to afford decent health insurance, and that they run and operate a small enterprise hiring themselves out in a plentiful "gig economy."

That is not the case for many. They are front-line workers with less fanfare than doctors, nurses, teachers, even grocery workers yet they provide care, direct support and many are immigrants, afraid to seek the care they need for fear of retaliation and false status reporting; thus risking everything, playing Russian roulette with their lives, the lives of their families, those they care for and going without vital care for themselves.

Caregivers that worked for families had to decide. When people in the home don't wear masks, they can't get immediate access to vaccines and they must be concerned with their health and that of their own families, often young children, in their home.

I resent the fact that most people suggest immigrants take jobs from people. Rarely are both Black people and White people the majority of applicants in the area where I live. They are not vying for these caregiving opportunities so that's a fallacy. The caregiving industry took a colossal and devastating impact, of low wages, no healthcare as I mentioned, and unpaid leave when they were sick (and they had to be very ill even to consider a day off,) they were just that dedicated often to great detriment to their health.) Families worried about losing their job having to time off in the caregiver's absence, and aging family caregivers gave the best they could but age, also compounded the issues of their ability to help. No one wanted to put their own safety at risk and what could anyone do? It was an impossible situation.

One thing you can't control is where your caregiver is going when they are away from you. These additional requirements made already tense situations and pressures worse. Who was going to ask about precautions being taken such as the numerously outed safety protocols of wearing masks, never mind being afraid to ask caregivers to wash their hands often, wearing the masks and reporting temperatures before arriving, when considering the climate, you were just happy they showed up at all.

No one had any bargaining power, any will to enforce when confronted by the thoughts of being stuck in bed if the caregiver didn't come for the day, no longer mattered or tugged on the heartstrings of those rendering care. Safety became paramount and people with disabilities were left. Even hospital personnel turned away people with disabilities on a belief system that still says lives with disabilities are not as important as our "typically functioning" peers.

It comes down to trust and to taking precautions to ensure the safety of others, but in the next chapter, I'll talk about emergency preparedness, and while most couldn't afford it, those with a few extra bucks to supplement their Medicaid or state-run programs, or pay a pretty penny outright, providing a caregiver in the home with an increase in their hourly wage, and thus make working in Covid times more palatable (and economical) for them to do so.

Money rules again. It appalled me to hear that in the height of Covid, if you required help, you could look to pay as much as $ 125.00 hourly for care. I guarantee Medicaid will not reimburse at such a high rate (they rarely reimburse caregiving expenses at all, but if they did,) it would not be at that amount.

In contrast, even in Northern Virginia, a very high-priced area, caregivers make just $ 13.60 hourly. They make even less in the southern part of the same state, at approximately $ 9.00 hourly. While I've primarily omitted any political speech in his book, this so-called "gray" area of Home and Community-Based Services (HCBS) is a part of the infrastructure of our lives. Caregivers permit me to work and support myself while earnings funds to put back into the economy and support the caregiver families who also contribute to the economy but provide people with disabilities opportunities to work and lead a dignifying life through this vital care. Where caregivers can't work to make a livable wage, where people with disabilities are not supported to work (who can and who desire to do so,) this creates an entire group of folks soon filing for entitlement programs and pulling on an overstretched system that can't meet all the current requests in the queue. With better wages and health insurance, the need for these programs could remain for those with the severest types of chronic conditions. It may be mitigated altogether by both groups becoming tax-paying individuals contributing to an economy in desperate need of recovery.

We are in crisis with our thoughts and actions (or inaction) around this subject. Covid pulled the covers off yet another area where we're remain so far behind.

TAKE ACTION ON CAREGIVING

- Build your confidence if you're unsure about how you personally can function as an employer. This applies to both self-advocates and their parents. Managing people is a skill that should be cultivated. Even if you're a small business owner, or perhaps even supervise thousands of people, managing the care of someone or yourself is vastly different. Remember that if you could make it on your own, you would, and that'd be great: you wouldn't need a caregiver, and that's wonderful. So many of us, however, have to really bite our tongues and choose our battles. Not everything is worth the fight or worth losing good people over.
- Before hiring anyone, assess your own needs. You need to be able to concisely convey what your needs are.
- Research and review what security precautions you should take. It may even be worth consulting with a residential security professional about potential modifications to the door locks, e.g. keypad entry.

When it comes to meeting individuals, screen folks over the phone first. I advise never meeting folks for the first time at your house.

- Become familiar with the laws in your particular state regarding setting up cameras and other recording and security measures, even live feeds to your cell phone for real-time monitoring. Some things are within your legal right to record unannounced; some things you'll have to disclose. In any case, research and follow the law in order to protect yourself in court, if it should ever come to that.

- Find out what you don't know. Begin to understand the ramifications, good and bad, of going into a nursing facility versus getting support/care in the home. Oh, and never assume that every kind of disability, ailment or setback automatically means nursing facility placement.

9 / EMERGENCY PREPAREDNESS

Key Takeaways

- If everything is going great right now, plan, plan,
  plan... then plan more. Unpreparedness can be
  more devastating than the issue itself. Planning
  now will mitigate deathly harm. In addition,
  planning can give you some peace of mind about
  what to do if confronted by certain challenges, or in
  the event that multiple challenges should befall you
  all at once.
- There are extreme worst-case scenarios, of course:
  weather-related, natural disaster-related,
  pandemic- related, all of which are complicated by
  socio-economic status deficits. For people with
  disabilities, though, these extremes do not have to
  feature at all in order for an event to qualify as an
  emergency. While the above examples are
  doubtless further complicated by the presence of
  one's disability, the fact remains that even a single

simple-seeming issue can disrupt our lives, becoming a disaster in and of itself.

- Despite all the planning in the world, you only have so much control. Try not to anticipate disaster or live a life of fear. Realize that planning is your best defense.

- The importance of having some additional funding stored away cannot be stressed enough. Folks with a few extra dollars saved can pay for the assistance they need, whereas those without access to funds often perish not only first but prematurely. While this may sound devastatingly dramatic, it is an historical fact.

- In the event of an emergency, the relationships you have or have not built will be revealed most in your time of pain and need. People you can count on in the worst of times are hard to come by. Remember this in all your relationships.

- DO NOT mess around in an emergency! Disability compounds things that are going wrong for able-bodied people. When the risk is high for your able-bodied friends, believe it's going to be a thousand percent worse for you!!

One of the experiences that worsened my anxiety the most was listening to all the calls coming into the CIL where I worked. With all the dire issues, emergencies and so on about which people would call in, together with the helplessness both they and I felt in having those conversations, I felt compelled to add this chapter. Some of these calls were, quite frankly, a kick in the pants. My inner response was so often that if you'd had called me earlier, if you had saved some funds, if, if, if… This response helped no one, least of all the person on the other end of the line who was, by this time, desperate for help.

Some examples of the things I've heard and helped to solve:

We're experiencing prolonged power outages; I'm on oxygen, and I use a power wheelchair.

I'm being evicted tomorrow.

I need to get to the hospital but it's not classified as an emergency.

I need to evacuate due to flooding (or fire, or mold spores). I use a wheelchair and I don't have a place I can go.

Listening to everything that was going wrong in peoples' lives just gave me all the worst-case scenarios that I could stand. The experience as a whole did heighten my own anxiety about everything for sure, but more importantly it helped me to picture worst-case scenarios for myself. As a result, I began to document issues so that I could also be of help to others going forward, having gathered the necessary data to mitigate adversity.

What I also learned through living and listening is that, whether they voice it or not, many people think there is nothing worse in life than having a disability. Dare I say that some people with disabilities become more daring because they think the worst possible injury has already happened? Wrong. Try physical disability with added head injury. And yes, some folks have all of those, but I'm not talking about that. I'm talking about how disability is not an "I can confront it all, I've already experienced the worst"-type deal. I'm disabled, yet I believe there are much worse things that can complicate my situation.

Living in poverty; racial inequality and discrimination; natural and manmade disasters; and on and on. Such things can hugely compound disability issues.

What is the contingency plan?

Who will help?

Who will you call?

How will you get what you need?

How will you pay for your unplanned needs?

At the risk of sounding like Bear Grylls: how will you get out alive?

First, on the natural, extreme weather and climate fronts, I've been fortunate enough to live in a relatively calm area as far as disasters are concerned. In 40 years, there's been only a small earthquake that did relatively little damage: my area is not known for earthquakes nor hurricanes. The power outage issues can be a bigger deal when you have significant essential equipment requiring power to run, from your power wheelchair to your bed to your transfer lift. (Many of these things can be charged up in advance, by the way, so there's another reason to charge your power chair and other devices every single night!)

Fires in California and Nevada have many folks seeking housing on the other side of the United States, refusing to remain in that cycle of constantly rebuilding their lives, sometimes three or four times over. Personally, I've never understood the whole rebuilding thing. If my house is knocked down once for any reason, peace out. The resources alone required to rebuild, with insurance only covering a portion of that expense at most - the displacement into temporary housing while your place is constructed – these factors and plenty more besides are enough of a deterrent for me. But I do understand that not everyone can move.

Where I live is not known for earthquakes or fires (knock on wood). Our most extreme weather event is record-setting snowfall. This is cold (duh), sometimes depressing, can often disrupt work and school, can be bad for folks who have trouble shoveling it, but it won't wipe out an entire neighborhood when it occurs. So far, the only issue has been a power outage that lasted almost three days. While that might not seem like a huge issue, if everything you use to go about your daily life is power dependent, from your wheelchair to your bed and even oxygen and ventilators for breathing, then it should be obvious that you can get into big trouble pretty fast. For me, emergency preparedness wasn't only related to natural disasters, but to these simpler things that are made into emergencies by the presence and prevalence of disability. Everything would be fine, *if it weren't for the disability,* and that is something you can't ever put on the shelf. Going north is an option, but those people obviously don't mind the cold and the snow.

Unfortunately, for those that need caregiving, heavy snow means you need someone to shovel it. In such situations, you'd be amazed at how quickly your caregivers start the no-show game - and you can hardly blame them, when state Departments of Transportation neglect the plowing of roads so badly that these highways are rendered both treacherous and hazardous for them to reach you in the first place. If a caregiver is injured because your walkways and footpaths aren't clear for them to reach your home, then you're looking at liability issues. Their own safety is paramount. Inviting someone to stay over a few nights is one option I have seen work in many circumstances, where the caregiver is willing and where space exists for them to stay and sleep comfortably.

But let's talk about an unfortunate, real-life, and devastating scenario. For an endless supply of these sad examples, we have to look no further than the reports that came out following hurricane Katrina in 2005. Here are just a few facts to refresh our memory:

- *Category 5 hurricane, affecting about 15 million people.*
- *Impacted 90,000 square miles of territory from central Florida to eastern Texas.*
- *Storm surge on the Mississippi coast reached 30 feet.*
- *The levees failed around Louisiana, having been originally designed only for storms up to Category 3.*
- *Produced 33 tornadoes.*
- *3rd largest hurricane ever recorded (#1 was Harvey in 2017; #2, Maria, also 2017.)*
- *Winds topped 175 mph during its peak.*
- *Cost approximately $160 billion.*
- *1800 people died.*

My point in mentioning these very tragic data points is to emphasize how disability complicates matters, and in an effort to help all of understand the total impact Katrina had.

If, as in many places, it's hard to get public transportation to go to the mall, or to hang out with your friends on a regular sunny summer day, how do you think transit services will look when everyone, including mass transit operators themselves, is looking out for their own safety and that of their families, and all public services have shut down?

If a social worker or case manager at a nonprofit schedules daily services for you, how will that change in the event of an emergency if they are landed with a 50-80 person caseload of people with disabilities who have similar needs, many of whom are prioritized above you?

Here's a snippet of one of the reports by the National Council on Disability that might drive my point home:

Almost immediately after Hurricane Katrina devastated the Gulf Coast, the National Council on Disability (NCD) estimated that there were roughly 155,000 people with disabilities over the age of 5 – or about 25 percent of the cities' populations – living in the three cities hardest hit by the hurricane: Biloxi, Mississippi; Mobile, Alabama; and New Orleans, Louisiana.[2] NCD urged emergency managers and government officials to recognize that for hurricane survivors with disabilities, their needs for basic necessities were "compounded by chronic health conditions and functional impairments... [which includes] people who are blind, people who are deaf, people who use wheelchairs, canes, walkers, crutches, people with service animals, and people with mental health needs."[3]

One story that could have ended so differently is that of Benilda Caixetta. Here's what the report said:

[On August 29] Susan Daniels called me to enlist my help because her sister-in-law, a quadriplegic woman in New Orleans, had been unsuccessfully trying to evacuate to the Superdome for two days. [...] it was clear that this woman, Benilda Caixetta, was not being evacuated. I stayed on the phone with Benilda for the most part of the day... She kept telling me she'd been calling for a ride to the Superdome since Saturday; but, despite promises, no one came. The very same paratransit system that people can't rely on in good weather is what was being relied on in the evacuation... I was on the phone with

Benilda when she told me, with panic in her voice "the water is rushing in." And then her phone went dead. We learned five days later that she had been found in her apartment dead, floating next to her wheelchair ... Benilda did not have to drown.

She didn't have to drown, but she did. This kind of story makes me so angry. As devastating as this story is, the anger is because it was *avoidable*. Despite my focus on disability complicating matters, it shouldn't have complicated things in this instance. It didn't have to be an insurmountable barrier. Disability is NOT insurmountable. Why wasn't this human seen?

This is, for me, more an issue of how we and everyone around us thinks about disability. It's about perception, and about a lack of problem solving skills all the parties involved, including Benilda herself, should have had. I'm not blaming the victim in any way, shape or form, but I must stress how people with disabilities can be their own problem solvers. While Benilda Caixetta is a victim, and while we have limited data in this particular scenario, here are some of the things I have a hard time with. First, I can't excuse the fact that she and her sister might have said the words, "someone, anyone come by with a couple of guys - firefighters, neighbors, police perhaps - that can transfer me into any kind of vehicle, a truck, a car, a forklift, who the hell cares, just get me outta here."

Could I leave my house as it fills with water? Water which in the confines of four walls can only rise and eventually kill me?

What will it cost me to go outside?

What will it cost me to remain inside?

Is there any visibility to be had by venturing out, where I

might encounter someone with a boat, or someone who is impelled to help me when confronted by my physical presence?

Is there any hill or area that's considered higher ground, and would someone see me if I got to that place?

Did whomever I was talking to perceive that only a wheelchair-equipped bus or lift-equipped vehicle might be something I could use to get out alive, to the exclusion of all other forms of transport: a taxi, school bus, private sedan, even a child's wagon?

I can't overstate this fact: I REFUSE TO SIT UP IN MY HOUSE AND DIE! Perhaps Benilda and her sister had come to a place where simply surviving was the only thing to do, even though waiting seemed the equivalent of dying.

I wonder how long she floated before she died? I wonder how far away her sister lived? I wonder, was there no other family or friend anywhere in the vicinity to attempt to go get her? I wonder if her sister would ask someone to drive her to get her sister? I wonder if the two women even believed dying was a strong probability?

In fact, I wonder whether Ms. Caixetta's home was already a sort of death trap where she could not enter and exit on her own. This question uncovers other problems that are devastating on their own, with or without the presence of an imminent disaster. *Why was she only found five days later?*

I wonder what others thought about her quality of life already?

This is the real issue, isn't it? For others looking in, sadly it is. You can research doctor Jack Kevorkian for more information on professionals that somehow arrive at notions that it's better to permit (even assist) a person to die than to help them to live. We have to confront the issue that some folks believe we aren't worth saving, and that resources would be better spent saving an ambulatory person whose intellectual functioning is considered "normal."

In Ms. Caixetta's case, there are of course more questions than answers. While I hate going there, I have to "go there" in my own life every single day, because of the things that make up who I am. We have to consider the stigma and the Intersectionality of all of the things that make up who we are. Ms. Caixetta may have been a minority, maybe not, but there are factors that suggest that she was. I don't know. Barring race and ethnicity, we do know she was a woman and that she had a disability. Would being of another race and/or gender have saved her? Would money to pay for private transportation and a plan to leave early have mattered to Ms. Caixetta?

Did the sister have funds to fly or drive in and be of more help, getting her sister out of there in time?

Were there any established relationships with caregivers? Did her neighbors know her at all?

In all of this, it's important not only to remember Ms. Caixetta's story and use it as a teaching moment, but to then go a step further and put yourself in her shoes.

What would you do?

A crazy idea to most but not me, if presented with a similar situation: could I help a family get into a hotel or Air B&B, paying for the shelter for all of us, and bartering for a place of safety and care for myself in exchange?

For people with disabilities, we have too many "doesn't haves" in life:

Doesn't transfer without assistance

Doesn't use smart devices or doesn't have access in the event of a power outage

Doesn't have emergency funds for a few nights' hotel stay

Doesn't have back-up power supply

Doesn't have back-up caregiver

Doesn't have an emergency duffle bag packed and ready to go at a moment's notice with everything one needs to survive two to three days (also called a "Bug Out" bag)

Doesn't have enough strong friendships or relatives living close by who care and will offer care or funds to help

Doesn't have their own accessible vehicle

Doesn't have reliable, accessible transit options in their community on any given day

Doesn't have shelters that are ADA compliant and are equipped to serve people with disabilities

Doesn't know where to rent a Hoyer lift

Doesn't have emergency medical suppliers who can expedite shipping supplies

Doesn't have enough funds

Doesn't have enough specialized transit or any at all

Doesn't have delivery options to stockpile some supplies to use ONLY in the event of an emergency

Doesn't have a single local men's, women's or family shelter that can accommodate a wheelchair user and his/her spouse and young children

Doesn't have any ASL interpreters at the shelter

Doesn't have any information in Braille

Doesn't have all emergency communications interpreted

Doesn't have back-up communication plan in the event of missing TTY machine

.   .   .

This list could go on forever. These day-to-day issues, whether emphasized by natural disaster, fire, flood or not, are realities that are going to happen regardless of whether or not you are prepared and stable enough to handle them.

Working in the disability advocacy field, there are dire emergencies and needs, some with some time to devote to them but most without a single hour to spare looking for help. The ability to think ahead can mean life or death for us. That's the bottom line. Whether you take a moment to read these reports or not, it doesn't mean disaster won't come for you in some other form for which you are also NOT prepared.

If I had to pick out three key factors from the scenarios I've illustrated, it would be difficult, because each situation is deeply unique and different based on the type of disability one has. For instance, if you're a diabetic, what are some of your concerns? Possibility of developing sores that you cannot see if those that assist in your care don't; ensuring you eat at the appropriate times; refrigeration for insulin. Can you get to the store to get a bag of ice? Do you have some icepacks sitting in your freezer right now that could buy you another eight to twelve hours of time in the event of a power outage? If you can't get to the store on your own, do you have a network of folks that could get on the phone or Internet to find someone who can? Your own emergency preparedness needs will be unique to you - and that's what you should be preparing for.

The three key factors outlined below stand out to me in disaster planning. These are just some examples that you can use in your own planning. I must also stress the need to write these things down or record them in some way. Would Ms. Caixetta have been able to think more clearly and strategize with her sister if she'd thought of options and recorded them somewhere ahead of time, i.e. before the water rushed in right before her very eyes? Panic only further complicates situations of stress, further preventing us from coming up with workable solutions.

Money - Financial data, which gained much more attention in the height of the pandemic, has outlined so many disruptors to our bottom line. Recent nationwide data showed that most Americans could not afford a $400 emergency without borrowing money from family and friends, or putting the cost on credit. (In all honesty, if you have some credit, that works too. We should not feel ashamed to have to use it: it is an emergency, after all). The point is that not many people have enough cash for anything, not even a $400 emergency. While that's unfortunate, let it be a clarion call to us all.

Secondly, *Availability* - hardly anyone is available for so many in times of urgent need, even first responders, at the exact same time during the height of an emergency. Think about it: there were not enough people to provide "specialized" transport assistance to Ms. Caixetta at the time she needed it, and her emergency also had a time sensitivity, to put it mildly.

Time to Prepare- If we thought the worst would happen, timing is key. Leaving early, going to the next state over, or somewhere not in the eye of the storm – somewhere that would receive at most some flooding.

In closing, I want to stress that this is not a chapter of blame. It's not about finger-pointing at all the shortcoming, limitations or lack of creative problem solving we may have as humans. It's not even about the unwillingness of so many services to come into compliance with the Americans with

Disabilities Act in order to accommodate people with disabilities who are in need. Those are the facts regardless. It is intended primarily as a wake-up call, to mitigate your own harm and injury. I also will note that during and after the hurricane, as with any natural disaster, people pulled together and solved problems: the cleanup efforts that commence, the surveying and repairing of damage. I believe this and it has been well documented. There are numerous articles and stories about communities coming together, helping one another; families and individuals, once strangers, taking in others, pooling resources and sharing their shelter, food, compassionate care and other resources to protect one another. The same processes were extended to people with disabilities, though too often only the tragedies such as Ms. Caixetta's story get highlighted.

This is also to note that even if you think you can't house someone with a disability, you are likely wrong. Granted, a person with a physical disability can't walk up to the third floor apartment - but could they be carried, if their life is in danger? Does anyone have a few wooden boards in their garage, to create a makeshift ramp and get a wheelchair user into the safety of their single family home, usually just a few steps? Can regular folks become caregivers where they haven't been and with zero experience?

The answer to all of these is yes: where they are willing and open, they can!

Finally, as important as my wheelchair is to me in giving me my freedom and independence and getting me everywhere I want and need to go, I can say that in the event of a mortal emergency, I won't hesitate to leave it. Transporting me might even injure me, or at least cause a few bruises, but I will be alive. I have to be real with my fellow friends with disabilities, too: as we know, sitting (or trying to, if you can't without lumbar and armrest supports) out of your customized wheelchair isn't fun, but bear in mind that equipment is replaceable: there is more to be manufactured for you when the dust settles. If our lives are at stake, we simply have to be willing to leave material things behind.

TAKE ACTION ON EMERGENCY PREPAREDNESS

- As I've mentioned, planning right now, while you're in a season of relatively smooth sailing is vital. CREATE A PLAN, then create a back-up plan for when things change at the last minute. Try to think of all worst-case scenarios - and what your response would be if they occurred all at the same time.
- Take a picture of your plan and send it to key friends and family – or better yet, create and save your plan in Google docs, making it accessible anywhere even if you lose your phone, computer, or Smart Tablet and have to use someone else's.
- Get a list from your pharmacy or make a list of medications you use, both names (generic and brand names) including dosage amounts. If displaced, another pharmacy can replace those meds for you.
- Do you know where to rent equipment if yours breaks down? Reach out to companies and ask for information to be sent to you on their services and

hours of operations. Bookmark these companies in your Google doc/plan.

- Build a file in a waterproof container with important information including these resources and your own essential paperwork. This might be something you can grab and go and, if flooded, may survive with you so you can get things back to normal.

- Sign up for local weather alert apps. These are free to use, and will alert you to impending weather-emergency information. Do not forget to change and update your apps whenever you relocate.

- Sign up with your local fire department. Many have programs that will put people with disabilities on a type of private registry (it's only accessible to the emergency managers) so that police, fire and rescue can have some basic details about you. In some states, they may be able to prioritize restoring power to your particular neighborhood or street more quickly, or conduct wellness checks more effectively knowing you and your situation. One of the issues I have personally had with this type of registry is the privacy policy and safeguards in place. In any case, it's important to ask questions about how the data will be used, to mitigate issues and to protect yourself. Consider, though, that the benefits may far outweigh any negative possibilities, especially if you live in an area prone to disaster.

- While now readily available, there was a time when not a single company could provide disability-friendly nationwide roadside assistance.

As more people with disabilities are becoming drivers, the need for someone to transport the accessible vehicle and the driver has increased. Some of those companies include

- Mobility Roadside Assistance - www.mobilityroadsideassistance.com,
- Dr. Handicap - www.dr.handicap.com, **https://adaautoclub**, and more resources are listed on my website

Many states have local boards that welcome your participation and service on them and include disaster and preparedness. The Partnership For Inclusive Disaster Strategies is the only organization of its kind dedicated to supporting local disability organizations. They offer a hotline that people with disabilities can call to obtain information and resources. For more information visit www.disasterstrategies.org

- In case of a power outage, or in the event that your home is no longer habitable for any reason, disability groups on Facebook, helpful neighbors on Nextdoor, and staff at Centers for Independent Living and Statewide Independence Living Councils can be lifelines. Ask them what they have done, ask them what groups they are in, and see if they share or have previously shared information in these forums. Start your research.
- Don't be afraid to discuss your needs with a friend or relative. The saddest thing about being a person with a disability can be that if you appear to have things figured out and seem inherently capable and resourceful already, no one sees the behind-the-

scenes of the immense work that had to be done in order to make every detail of your life happen. Because of this, outsiders often assume that you don't need assistance, or that if you do, someone you know will magically arrive to help you - even that you will simply figure it out. Tell, share, then demonstrate how they can be of assistance. You may find that many more folks than you thought are willing to help you: they are simply unsure of how best to offer support.

- Wherever possible, know what things cost and make a plan to save those emergency funds. A week-long hotel stay is one cost, but what about paying a caregiver - or even a support specialist, for children and adults with intellectual and developmental disabilities? What's your plan if you're not receiving any home and community-based services in your state through Long Term Care insurance or Medicaid and Medicare based programs? While it may not cost you anything to live in your home (beyond your rent/mortgage in this example), e.g. supports, keep in mind everything you have gradually figured out and adapted in your setting and how comparatively smoothly it now works and flows. You cannot always replicate that same accessibility in a home away from home. This could be a rental, or a government-issued trailer, or some other temporary shelter. Another issue highlighted by the report on Hurricanes Katrina and Rita, by the National Council on Disability, was that the Red Cross's inventory of possible housing did not take into the account the needs of displaced persons with varying abilities, nor where to rent any special equipment beyond a standard manual wheelchair they may have already possessed. In a word, you may be able to get shelter, but it may require more equipment or extra supplies. Plus, consider that you may have to eat out, often up to two weeks or more - or eat lean for a few days, if you cannot cook your own food in this inaccessible housing situation. Monies may also be needed for specialized transport, Durable Medical Equipment, replacement of ruined supplies, extra medication, clothes and personal care items.

- Does your family know what your after-life plans are and what you desire? Facing the pandemic last year, many parents got the push they needed to finally set up proper documents for the care of their children/spouse, etc, in the event of their own demise. We all need to create preparedness plans for our families. These plans should include power/s of attorney, healthcare directives, and wills in place, so that it's as easy as possible for those left behind to implement whatever preferences you have.

- It's a smart idea to identify local shelters that are equipped to house people with special needs in the event of a disaster. Don't be afraid to call and ask them: are they able to accommodate, and if so, how?

- A "bug out" bag list and a few videos of where I learned what exactly a "bug out" bag is, are available at my website.

A longer list of Emergency Kit Supplies can be found at the website resources we've listed to assist you, but here is a short list to get started:

- Photocopies of important documentation such as health insurance policies, ID cards, and medical alert information.
- Copies of all prescription drugs that your child takes and contact information for doctors and pharmacies in case you need an emergency refill.
- Special instructions for administering medication if someone must provide assistance and the primary usual person is not available.
- Extra batteries for medical devices such as hearing aids, breathing machines and transport lifts.
- Your wheelchair battery charger if you use a power wheelchair or scooter.
- A patch kit to repair tires on a wheelchair or scooter in an emergency.
- A two-week supply of medical care items such as needles, bandages, etc.
- Cooler and ice packs for any medications that must be kept cold.
- Masks, gloves, blankets, and towels, paper towels, tissues.
- A back-up supply of special dietary foods and supplements.
- A lightweight manual wheelchair to use as a back-up in the event a power chair dies or fails, or if you need to be transferred and then transported.
- A "grab and go", also called a "bug out" bag, of items

that will keep your child calm - such as toys that he
or she likes, or a favorite book.

- Extra food and supplies for service animals.
- A power adapter that can be plugged into the car
  for any electronic communication devices, e.g.
  smart phones and tablets.
- Flashlights, batteries.
- Portable Radio.
- Phone chargers.
- Meal kits - small meal packs that do not require
  refrigeration; canned goods, including tuna,
  chicken, ham, beef, beef jerky; pasta, lentils, cereal,
  granola bars, oatmeal, peanut butter, nuts and
  crackers, chips and cookies, water, individual juice
  boxes, apple sauce...
- Matches / lighters.
- A more comprehensive lists of items to include can
  be found at www.fema.org and www.redcross.org

At your leisure, consider reading the in-depth reports
compiled in the wake of recent devastating events and world
pandemics, to better meet the needs of people with disabilities
in the future. One such report is linked below:

- See National Council on Disabilities report: ***The
  Impact of Hurricanes Katrina and Rita
  on People with Disabilities: A Look Back
  and Remaining Challenges***
- Centers for Disease Control (CDC) COVID -19
  Infectious Diseases as it pertains to special needs
  populations and people with disabilities,

information portal. Research indicates that many people with disabilities are thankfully NOT especially prone to COVID 19 when compared with other groups of people; however, there are a number of circumstances that contradict this statement. The CDC talks about precautions for people with disabilities, both generally and specifically pertaining to group home settings, homeless populations, and people in nursing and immediate care facilities. Such communal settings can potentially attract more diseases and germs due to the quality of care in these institutions and the high overturn of personnel in these settings. See ***Covid 19 CDC Precautions for People with Disabilities***

THE PARENT - DISABLED CHILD MANIFESTO

Whatever prognosis the doctor said, after you leave him or her, decide to move on to your next step mentally. You're not the first, and you won't be the last to receive less than stellar news. I hate to sound chastising, but doctors indeed know what they see. They use some historical data to deliver to you what statistics say, "now this is, and how it's going to go for you..." and you consider and gobble up every word, believing and buying into the fact that your situation will be exactly like those of others.

I don't find many (if any) doctors who report on those surprising stories that share with you those magical patients that beat all the odds to sway you away and maybe, inspire you to a path of hope so far from their dismal reporting.

Some things you can do, reading this book for one, great job! Here's a type of contract I'd like you to make for yourself and with your special needs child. Consider this your marching orders. Why not have a conversation with your child (depending on the age and intellectual acuity) that these are the ways and means you will both strive to treat each other. I'm confident these will be truly enlightening and possibly, uplifting conversations.

1. Dignity and respect - let's agree that due to disability, I'm not somehow less than everyone else. I may have less physically (or intellectually) to work with, but at every stage, I'm a human being first. People will treat me how YOU have treated me. They will see our interactions and make judgments and perceptions about what our relationship is like. When I'm alone with them or out in this world, the respect and dignity you gave me will influence how they respond to my needs and wants and overall treatment of me and how I see them and their role in my life.

2. Treatment from Others - If you don't have a favorable outlook about my life, how can you expect others to have an optimistic view of me and the capabilities of people with disabilities in general?

3. Renew your mind - Get outside yourself to ask other parents, more than one, gathering lots of varied and diverse perspectives and ways to cope with the issues I have. If you don't see anyone like you and me, start your group and watch people come in waiting for you to share your knowledge and to build on expertise while forming a community around similar shared experiences.

4. Speak Up! - People are going to say all kinds of things about our family. You can handle it, and it will be

5. Let me participate! I'm going to want to do things, and instead of saying you don't know how you're not sure, you have to develop an attitude of "you can make it happen." I will learn this directly from

YOU. I'll either wither and die at every bout of adversity and turn into a depressed, little sad kind of human being, or watching you confront things on my behalf will motivate me never to give up and to keep trying. I'll start to think creatively about what I can do to permit my participation. A can-do attitude says: "We can do this." Advocacy, fundraising, talking to people and authorities that might scare you to death will be the case, but you can do it. When you relegate everyone to put their pants on one leg at a time like the rest of us, you level the playing field and remove the scary parts that might deter you. Everything can start with a conversation, and you can't be afraid to have them. Within this same directive, I realize that I will want to try new things, travel, use Metro, and all the other regular things my "typically functioning peers" are doing. You will have to let go, maybe the first few times you can follow me or find a peer to accompany me and help look out for my well-being and safety, but I need autonomy to do what I feel like I can do. It would help if you relaxed the reigns a little bit, especially as I age and desire to grow and learn. Progression is healthy for me, and this is not about you at all. It's about my coming of age, growing up, and finding my way through this thing called life, but it will require a great deal of patience on your part as you reckon with the changes I'll go through into adulthood.

6. Get me out of here! Realize when some things aren't a good fit; however, do question and challenge me first. Some things I'm crying wolf over

but some things it is time to exit. When I say it's time to go, wait rather than catering to my every need every time something doesn't work. Let's have a conversation about why it's not working and see if we can first improve my attitude about it and processes and outcomes.

7. Keep your autonomy and, for God's sake, practice self-care - A whole lot of self-sacrifice going on to the point of exhaustion, resentment, self-neglect, hurt feelings, and bouts of crying into your coffee as you sit alone in the car. Push back and ask people to chip in. When I've got my own thing as a healthy, thriving adult now, what on earth are you going to do with yourself that's just for you? What is something that is a passion that you love to do regardless of what others say? Don't wait until you're "done" rearing me to get your life back; always keep a piece of that life front and center and take time for yourself.

8. You don't know everything; admit it (yes, okay, fine, silently to yourself, when alone, in the dark.) It's okay to admit what you did or didn't do might not have been the right call, but you won't know until you make any call at all. You cannot become paralyzed by analysis and overthinking everything. Make a decision, even if later, you must admit, perhaps it wasn't the right choice.

9. My way... is sometimes okay (as long as I don't fatally injure myself) - At times, we let some folks, say your husband, for instance, get away with some of his questionable parenting skills? It's not the way you would have done something, but it is a way to

do it, his way, my way, and still, the job is complete. Sometimes my way won't be pretty, it probably won't be all that efficient, but there are concessions that both of us are going to have to make, not to mention doing it on my own, in my way, is dignifying and respectful and permits me to do it at my own pace. If it takes all day, let me do it; let me try. Be patient enough to let me keep trying and not only let me try but be encouraging as I do.

10. Please don't compare me to my siblings or anyone else, for that matter. The thief of joy is comparison, and sitting around counting, marking days as you look at my siblings or other families in our circles robs every one of their path and story. None of these bouts of comparison rituals is helping me find my way or build a healthy sense of self, strong self-esteem, and autonomy. It's certainly not making you feel any better. It's robbing you (and me) of all the awesome things I can do at my own pace, at my own time when I'm permitted to do so.

If we can remember these things, we will get through everything together, and we will feel a real sense of accomplishment. We must have each other's back no matter what, and we must work together, always to accomplish all of our hopes and dreams.

IS IT YOUR TURN?

Please keep reading to find out how to join us and tell your stories, too.

As I mentioned, this book has been a long journey, but one built on my passion for sharing stories, relaying helpful information and resources, encouraging others, and building community. All of it has been a labor of love. I can't seem to let this writing thing go. To realize the original dream of this project that I talked about at the beginning, where there are multiple contributors with disabilities, I'd like to extend this invitation to you to help me write Volume 2. When you see the cover of this book, it says "Volume 1," so there's gotta be a sequel, right? Who knows when it will end? I mean, the Fast and the Furious franchise is still going strong; why not us?

Below, I cover some guidelines for contributors to keep in mind. Please consider choosing a topic and penning your personal story on any topic you feel has a beautiful lesson and will appeal to others with disabilities. There is a ton more information and tips to be gleaned from our collective experiences.

Please follow the same format I have in this book, with:

1. *Key Takeaways* - can be generated from your actual chapter, things in the chapter, or additional components you may not have touched on in the chapter.

2. *Chapter Body* - Your story, how it did it happen, what happened? What did you learn? How did you confront the issue, and what would you like others to take from your experience? Whether good or bad, what can readers take from you to make an impact on their own lives and the lives of their families, caregivers and practitioners, and service providers?

3. *Take Action* - sum up the chapter with bulleted tips and motivating direct action steps others can take to deal with the very subject matter you are writing about. Include what you did or what you wished you might have done to improve the trajectory of the outcomes. Use evidence-based solutions wherever possible.

Any contributions will remain the author's original work. All chapters selected for publication will receive a small monetary stipend for your time and should be edited before submission. Any chapters that we find valuable but may not fit the book, or the book has reached its content limit goals, can be featured on the blog if you permit its release and sharing on our site. There will be no compensation for Blog features, only the exposure and promotion on our site and social media for the author. Feel free to pitch your topic before actual writing if you'd like some support, feedback, but we're sure many desire to have and are in need of the information you deem worth sharing.

Below are just a few topics we'd like to discuss next and get you started on your ideas; however, keep in mind that if it's not listed here and you have something you'd like to discuss, that is fine, we welcome it. Please submit what you want to write about and what you think is a good fit, and then let us have a look.

- Purchasing a wheelchair, other Durable Medical Equipment, or vehicle
- Dating and Relationships
- Finding Love and Marriage
- End-of-Life Planning
- Entrepreneurship and Side Hustles
- Family planning
- Parents perspectives welcome (working with others on behalf of your child) with a disability
- Parenting with a disability
- IVF, Adoption, and Surrogates
- Healthcare and managing illness, chronic conditions
- Health and wellness
- Quitting Full-Time Employment for Disability Benefits
- Living alone, living on your own, living with others
- Making Life Work
- Home modifications and building from the ground up; unique home arraignments

Are you ready? Please send all inquiries or submissions to: hello@traceegarner.com. Please expect to hear from us within 10-12 weeks.

GLOSSARY

INDEX / Glossary

The listing does not imply endorsement. All programs, websites, individuals, companies, and organizations that we will list should be thoroughly researched, references checked, and precautions taken before taking advice or using any services provided from the list of agencies and organizations Some terms are not necessarily in the text but may be defined for clarity or informational purposes only.

Assistive Technology Loan Fund Authority (ATLFA) - [See Newell Fund] in Virginia, though versions of the program may exist in other states and be called by a different name; provide low or zero-interest loans and grants to people with disabilities their family's. Funds received can be used to pay for durable medical equipment, vehicle or home modifications, etc.
   Adaptive recreation *p.*

Adaptive fitness - (See Chapters on Physical Health, Recreation)

Barrier-free lift - (see also Hoyer lift, also called patient transport lift) - a type of transferring device used to hoist the patient up from their chair to transfer them to another device, e.g., a bed, commode, or bathtub. Hoyer lifts are portable and often break down into two or more parts; Barrier Free machines are usually stationary and mounted into the ceiling or wall or one's bathroom, bedroom, or other living areas. Hoyer lifts can be rented from local equipment companies for travel, vacations in many states.

Bowling assistance ramp - (sometimes called bowling ramp) p. 112

Careers and the Disabled (magazine) — Established in 1986, the magazine is the first and only publication explicitly focused on employment topics related to people with disabilities. An Equal Opportunity Publication. https://www.eop.com/mags-CD.php

Caregiving p. 123; (also called Personal Care Assistant, Home Health Aid, Home Health Care Worker, Personal Care Attendant, Personal Assistant) p.

Center for Medicaid and Medicare Services (CMMS) p. 83

Centers for Independent Living (CILs)- Federally funded nonprofit agencies that offer services to people with disabilities from a peer-based support model. 400 centers nationwide.

Climate emergencies p. 100

Developmental delay - (also called Developmental disability) a group of conditions due to an impairment in physical ability, intellectual capacity for learning, language processing or behaviors. (Often persons diagnosed with a developmental disability prior to the age of 22 can qualify for certain programming services, funding, and aide that those who experienced injuries and other disabilities later in life, cannot.

Diversability (*magazine*) *p.*

https://diversabilitymagzine.com/

Emergency Preparedness - (See chapter 9) p. 141

Employment - (See chapter 2) p. 1

Guttman, Ludwig p. 112

Home Automation Consultant - (also knowns as SMART Home Specialist) — p. 104 Usually, a licensed or certified consultant assists homeowners/renters with identifying suitable security automation tools and enhancements to purchase and install. These enhancements help things run more accessibly and efficiently in the home (and can be operated through touch or voice activation, and often from your Smartphone or other technology). There is not much data to suggest these consultants are versed in disability-specific accommodations. However, including a PT/OT or Rehabilitation Specialist could be one way to ensure the person's needs are met and that workable solutions fit most appropriately.

Home and Community-Based Services (HCBS) —*p.* 135

Housing — (*See chapter 6*) *p.* 80

Hoyer lift — p. 70 (See also Barrier Free Lift, also called patient transport lift) - a type of transferring device used to hoist the patient up from their chair, to transfer them to another device, e.g., a bed, commode, or bathtub. Hoyer lifts are portable and often break down into two or more parts for easy transport in the trunk of a car, or other vehicle; Barrier Free machines are usually stationary and mounted into the ceiling or wall or one's bathroom, bedroom, or other living areas. Hoyer lifts can be rented from local equipment companies for travel, vacations in most states.

Hurricanes — p. 144 (see also natural disasters, climate emergencies)

    Hurricane Katrina — p. 146 (y. 2005)

    Hurricane Rita — p. 146 (y. 2005)

    Individualized Education Plan (IEP) — p. 15

Created through a team of invested folks, parents, teachers, therapists, school administrators, guardians/caregivers) surrounding children and youth with disabilities. This plan is a federally binding document holding members to a specific course of education supports for the child's instruction and learning. ***Mainstream Instruction*** — p. 7 (classroom education vs. self-contained) a mainstream classroom is a general education classroom. Mainstreaming means putting kids with an IEP in the general education classroom for some or most of the day. An inclusion classroom is a general education classroom that has some students who receive special education.

Loan closet — p. 91; A warehouse, or other multipurpose space that houses Durable Medical Equipment such as manual and power wheelchairs, walkers/rollators, canes, crutches, chair lifts, hospital beds, and Hoyer lifts) for the unrestricted (and free) use of by people with disabilities. Most loan closets are run by CIL's or other nonprofit or government agencies such as Adult Protective Services (APS) through your local Area Agency on Aging (AAA or sometimes referred to as AoA's)

Medicaid Waiver Program, (Also called the Commonwealth Coordinated Care Plus (CCC+) program (in Virginia) formerly the Elderly and Disabled Consumer Director (EDCD) Waiver Program. Medicaid programs can provide people with disabilities direct-care, home caregiver support to pay for caregivers in the home and some other technologies to support the person with a disability, daily living activities.

Mental Health — (See chapter 3)

Muscular Dystrophy (MD) — p. 53 A degenerative neuromuscular disease often had at birth but diagnosed in toddlers, but can be diagnosed later in adolescence, and adulthood.

Amyotrophic Lateral Sclerosis (ALS) — a form of Muscular Dystrophy (also called Lou Gehrig's Disease)

Muscular Dystrophy Association (MDA) — a national organization dedicated to supporting families who have a child with one or more of the 45+ types of MD and conducting research to mitigate the disease from birth.

National Arc, The — national advocacy organization catering to those with Intellectual and Developmental disabilities.

Natural disaster - p. 100

(NCHPAD) National Center on Health, Physical Activity and Disability — p. 114 - www.nchpad.org

Newell Fund - (see also Assistive Technology Loan Fund Authority (ATLFA)) p. - in Virginia. However, versions of the program may exist elsewhere (and be called by a different name), provide low or zero-interest loans to people with disabilities and their family's to pay for durable medical equipment, vehicle or home modifications, etc.

Paralympics — p. 111

Partners in Policymaking (PIP) Program — p. 2; A 9-month leadership training program usually held in the state capitol for parents of children with disabilities, and self advocates to learn about laws, policies and legislation as it relates to disability advocacy and speaking up for ones self.

Parasport — p. 113

Physical Health — (See chapter 4) p. 49

Paratransit — p. 71

Physical education (PE) — p. 106

Policygenius — p. 102

Recreation — p. 107

self-contained classes — Definition: the term "self-contained classroom" refers to a classroom where a special education teacher is responsible for the instruction of all academic subjects. The classroom is typically separated from general education classrooms but often still maintained in a subsection of a typical neighborhood school.

Silva, Derek — *p.* 103

SMART Home consultants (*see also Home Automation Consultant*) *p.* 104

Support services (SS) — different types of support services for youth and adults can be paid with local benefits, such as Medicaid, or can be contracted directly paying out of pocket. SS may also include Caregiver Support and Behavioral Support programs.

Direct Support Services — professionals usually experienced in child development, who work with people with disabilities in school, work, home settings to provide support and instruction on daily life skills, independent living support and other types of services that promote the wellbeing, autonomy of individuals with disabilities; many often work in the home setting or a residential facility, congregate home or group home settings.

Workforce Recruitment Program (WRP) — *p.* 24; an often paid, summer internship program focused on recruiting students with disabilities and placing them into federal government positions for learning and skill development.

Ullman, Shawn — p. 81

Youth Leadership Forum (YLF) — *p.* 2; a weeklong advocacy training program in many states where juniors and seniors with disabilities visit and stay on campus (usually) for one week, attend classes, build skills, and learn about advocacy while strengthening their leadership style.

ABOUT THE AUTHOR

A LITTLE HELP FROM MY FRIENDS. . .
EXPERIENCE

A staunch disability advocate, Tracee Garner, has been described as a force of nature. Innovative, intuitive, and creative approach to solving complex access issues with a dose of attitudinal barriers with heartfelt ways to reach the audience whose mind needs to change. All of this within a world that still is mainly inaccessible for people with disabilities. In her writing, she uses her words and voice to champion the rights of people with disabilities and the unserved and underserved populations. In this topical bible about issues that all people with disabilities will face, if they haven't already, she is assisting her fellow compatriots with advice, tips, and insight on a vast array of her experiences. She has completed many of those experiences, from obtaining fulfilling, gainful employment to the challenges of finding competent mental health practitioners and the complexity of needs on behalf of every disability type with some universal principles that relate to all of us as human beings first. In this book, Tracee shares the good, bad, and hilarity of situations with hopes to help other people with disabilities move ahead in their own lives. Whether a newly disabled person or a veteran, her ideas and support in helping you navigate potential pitfalls in "gimpy life" are clear and doable. She's lived through the issues she speaks of and gives accessible advice and tips to help you power chair through.

Tracee Garner is a best-selling author of more than fourteen fiction and nonfiction titles, a speaker, book coach, and course creator with a wealth of knowledge. A native of Virginia, Tracee currently resides in a suburb of the DC metro area with her family. She enjoys writing, day excursions throughout the cityscapes, and helps aspiring writers finish writing, publish and market their books. Diagnosed with Muscular Dystrophy at the age of two, Tracee has used a wheelchair since elementary school and has been an advocate for people with disabilities since her teen years. Visit www.TraceeGarner.com for fiction titles, courses, and teaching resources, and www.Garner-Solutions.com for disability-related topics and themes, and her blogs. Enjoy the accompanying podcast also on both sites for this excellent new book.

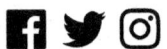